WINDY DRYDEN was born in London in 1950. He has worked in psychotherapy and counselling for over 25 years, and is the author or editor of over 100 books, including *Overcoming Jealousy* (Sheldon Press, 1998) and *Ten Steps to Positive Living* (Sheldon Press, 1994). Dr Dryden is Professor of Counselling at Goldsmiths College, University of London.

Overcoming Common Problems Series

Selected titles

A full list of titles is available from Sheldon Press,
36 Causton Street, London SW1P 4ST and on our website at
www.sheldonpress.co.uk

Overcoming Common Problems

How to Accept Yourself

Dr Windy Dryden

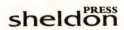

First published in Great Britain in 1999

Sheldon Press
36 Causton Street
London SW1P 4ST

British Library Cataloguing-in-Publication Data

A catalogue record for this book is available
from the British Library

ISBN-13: 978–0–85969–942–6
ISBN-10: 0–85969–942–0

3 5 7 9 10 8 6 4 2

Typeset by Deltatype Ltd, Birkenhead, Merseyside
First printed and bound in Great Britain by
Biddles Ltd, King's Lynn, Norfolk
Reprinted and bound in Great Britain by
Ashford Colour Press

Contents

Introduction

There are many books on the market which offer to help you to improve your self-esteem. This book is different. I am not going to help you to improve your self-esteem. Rather, I am going to outline ways in which you can develop self-acceptance. No, I'm not splitting hairs, being pedantic or just playing with words. In my view, self-esteem and self-acceptance are different concepts, and I regard the latter to be far healthier for you than the former.

Are you intrigued? I hope so. But I will not discuss these points here in the introduction. Rather, I will take this opportunity to invite you to read this book and embark with me on a journey that is arduous, but fulfilling: the journey towards self-acceptance.

1

Do You Have a Problem with Low Self-esteem?

Not all psychological problems can be traced to low self-esteem (or what I refer to in this book as self-depreciation), but a lot can. This is why I have written this book. However, problems with self-depreciation come in many different guises and in this opening chapter I will consider the different facets of this debilitating attitude towards yourself.

The presence of self-depreciation in common emotional problems

In this section, I will consider eight common emotional problems and discuss where self-depreciation fits into each problem. I do want to stress at the outset that I am not saying that self-depreciation is the only factor present in each problem, nor that it is necessarily the main factor involved, although it can be. Rather, I want to show that self-depreciation crops up in many problems and that if you want to lead a psychologically healthy life, self-depreciation will significantly interfere with your aspirations. Dealing productively with self-depreciation is important, therefore, if you want to overcome common emotional problems, and if you wish to be psychologically healthy. So let me consider the common emotional problems one by one and show where self-depreciation fits in.

Anxiety

When you are anxious you consider that you are facing some kind of threat. There are, in fact, two types of anxiety: discomfort anxiety and ego anxiety. In ego anxiety, if the threat materializes then you will depreciate yourself in some way. Typical ego-based threats concern the prospect of doing poorly at a task (in which case you will consider yourself to be a failure or incompetent), the prospect of being criticized (in which case you will consider yourself to be worthless) or the prospect of being disapproved (in which case you will consider yourself to be an unlikeable person). For example, Jamie was anxious about speaking in public and tried to avoid doing so whenever possible. On the occasions when he had to speak in public he was anxious in case he said something foolish in which case he would regard himself as a fool.

Depression

When you feel depressed you consider that you have lost something very important to you or that you have failed at an important task. Typical self-depreciations in depression are: 'I am a failure', 'I am useless' and 'I am unlovable'. For example, Fiona became depressed when her longstanding boyfriend ended their relationship. She regarded this loss as evidence that she was unlovable and that no one else would want her.

Guilt

You tend to feel guilty about doing something wrong, not doing the right thing or hurting someone's feelings. The most common self-depreciation in guilt is: 'I am a bad person'. For example, Bill, a single man of 40 who had lived with his parents all his life, became very guilty when he left home because he regarded himself a rotten person for hurting their feelings.

Shame

You tend to feel ashamed when you fall very short of some ideal or when you have revealed an inadequacy or defect in public. In particular, you think that others who witness your behaviour will look down on you, ignore you or turn away from you in disgust. Typical self-depreciations in shame include: 'I am insignificant', 'I am defective' or 'I am repulsive'. For example, Josie considered that she was ugly and wore make-up to hide the wrinkles underneath her eyes. If other people saw her wrinkles she predicted that they would feel disgusted and she would consider herself to be a repulsive person as a result.

Unhealthy jealousy

When you experience unhealthy jealousy, you consider that your relation-ship with your partner, for example, is threatened by a rival for your partner's affections. Typical self-depreciations in unhealthy jealousy include: 'I am unlovable', 'I am no good' and 'I am nothing if I lose my relationship'. Harriet felt unhealthily jealous whenever she saw her boyfriend, Michael, talking to an attractive woman, because she inferred that Michael was interested in having a relationship with the other woman which would mean that she, Harriet, was worthless.

Hurt

When you experience feelings of hurt you consider that you have been treated in a way that you do not deserve by a significant other who you do not expect to treat you in this manner (e.g. that the other person has betrayed your trust). Typical self-depreciations in hurt include: 'I am unlovable', 'I am of no account as a person', 'I am insignificant'. Donald experienced hurt when his best friend forgot to send him a birthday card, taking this as evidence that his best friend did not care for him as much as he cared for his friend. If this was true, Donald reasoned that it would prove that he was of less importance as a person, not only to his friend, but to himself.

Unhealthy envy

When you experience unhealthy feelings of envy, you focus on the fact that someone possesses something, such as a desired characteristic or object, that you do not have, and you hold the belief that this proves that you are less worthy than the other person. For example, Janice experienced unhealthy feelings of envy towards Mary, an acquaintance of hers, who got a first-class honours degree whereas she only got a lower second. Janice concluded that this meant that she was less worthy than Mary, although as often happens in unhealthy envy she disguised this from herself and set about denigrating Mary instead.

Unhealthy anger

When self-depreciation is a major feature of unhealthy anger, you consider that another person has put you in a bad light and you think that this proves that you are unworthy or bad. Instead of feeling depressed, however, you feel angry towards the person who you think has made you feel badly about yourself. This is known as ego-defensive anger. You are defending your ego against attack from another person by attacking that person with your anger. For example, Barry made himself unhealthily angry at his wife when she criticized him for being thoughtless. Deep down, Barry agreed with the criticism, but because he thought that this proved that he was worthless he got angry at his wife for making him feel this way. I should point out that this complicated psychological process normally occurs extraordinarily quickly outside the awareness of the person who is angry.

What we depreciate ourselves about

Let me shed a slightly different light on self-depreciation by considering what we tend to put ourselves down about. In doing so, I will describe the most common effects that self-depreciation has on the way we act and on the way that we tend to view life. In particular, I will consider the effects of self-depreciation on our relationships with other people.

Before I consider what we most commonly put ourselves down about, I want to make an extremely important point, one which forms the core of this book and one which I will repeatedly stress as the book unfolds. It is this: events on their own do not cause us to depreciate ourselves. Rather, self-depreciation is an attitude of mind that we bring to these events which results in us feeling badly about ourselves. This does not mean that the events of our lives are unimportant in understanding self-depreciation. This is certainly not the case, in that we normally do not put ourselves down in a vacuum. But these events contribute to rather than directly cause our feelings of inadequacy, worthlessness and the like. Our beliefs about ourselves largely determine our feelings about ourselves. Remember this point as you read on.

Having stressed the central importance of our beliefs about ourselves, let me discuss the most common areas in life in which we depreciate ourselves and the most common effects of such self-depreciation.

Failing to achieve an important goal

When you fail to achieve something that is important for you to achieve and you put yourself down for your failure, you tend to equate your failure in this area with your failure as a person. As I will discuss more fully in the next chapter, this is an example of you defining yourself according to your behaviour. If you fail you think that this means that you are a failure as a person. Once you have defined yourself as a failure, you then tend to give up pursuing your valued goal because you think that it is not worth you exerting further effort since, as you see it, there is very little or no chance of success. In addition, once you regard yourself as a failure then you tend to access memories of past failures and find it increasingly difficult to think of times when you have been successful. Even when you can remember times when you have been successful, your view of yourself as a failure affects how you think of these successes. Thus, you tend to attribute these successes to luck rather than to your own abilities.

When you consider yourself to be a failure for having failed to achieve an important goal, you tend to avoid other people whom you see as being successful. If you are unable to avoid such people you try to steer the conversation away from areas where they have been successful and you have failed. Sometimes you compensate for your sense of being a failure by mixing with people whom you do not find threatening (e.g. people who have failed to achieve much in life or people who have achieved less than you). Thus, you try to manage your relationships with people so that you are not reminded of being a failure.

Acting incompetently (in public or private)

When you act incompetently in public or in private and you depreciate yourself for this, you again equate your self with your behaviour. For example, if you act foolishly you tend to think of yourself as a foolish person. If this happens in the presence of others you experience a strong tendency to withdraw from others, and if it happens in private you try to avoid being with others who may find out about your behaviour. When you consider yourself to be a fool for acting foolishly, for example, then you overestimate the extent to which other people who witnessed or found out about what you did will disapprove of you and how long they will remember your foolish behaviour. You also overestimate the negativity of their response to you. Thus, when you depreciate yourself for your incompetent behaviour you think that others will either look down on you or turn away from you. You certainly don't expect others to empathize or be compassionate towards you, and if they do show such responses you tend to think that they are only doing so out of pity.

Breaking your ethical/moral code

When you break one of your ethical or moral codes and you condemn yourself for doing so, you tend to view yourself as a bad or rotten person for doing so. If what you did was bad then in your mind you are a bad person. In thinking this way about yourself, you tend to want to hurt or punish yourself in some way. This may take the form of a passive punishment where you refrain from doing anything to enjoy yourself, or it may involve you actively punishing yourself where you destroy something that you value. You may even experience a strong desire to hurt yourself physically. If this is the case, especially if you act on these destructive impulses, then I suggest that you seek appropriate professional help for you need more assistance than I can offer you in this book. If transgressing your ethical or moral code has involved you hurting others, then when you condemn yourself for your actions you will either beg others for forgiveness or do far too much in the way of offering reparation. Even when you go 'over the top' in your efforts to make up to the other person for having hurt or harmed them, feeling that you are a rotten person for breaking your code, you think deep down that you are beyond forgiveness, such is the nature of your badness as as person. Thus, you are suspicious of the other's forgiveness and think that you do not deserve any understanding that they may show you. If you are religious, when you think that you are bad for breaking your code then you consider that God will not forgive you and that you will go to hell when you die.

Being criticized

When you are criticized and you put yourself down in the face of this criticism, you again tend to overgeneralize in one or more ways. For example, if someone criticizes you for being mean with money, there are a number of possibilities:

1 The person is criticizing you for being mean with money: this is a fair criticism, but she does not depreciate you for this.
2 The person is criticizing you for being mean with money: this is a fair criticism, and she does depreciate you for this.
3 The person is criticizing you for being mean with money: this is an unfair criticism, but she does not depreciate you for this.
4 The person is criticizing you for being mean with money: this is an unfair criticism, and she does depreciate you for this.

You can depreciate yourself in all these circumstances, but when you do put yourself down in the face of criticism, you are likely to think that the conditions outlined in the second scenario hold. In other words, you tend to think that the person's criticism is fair when it may be unfair and that the person is depreciating you when this may not be the case.

When you are particularly prone to depreciating yourself in the face of criticism you anticipate being criticized in the absence of available evidence that this might be the case. In addition, you may develop a defensive attitude and immediately deny any criticism that you may receive without considering whether the criticism has any merit. Behaviourally, when you are prone to depreciating yourself in the face of criticism, you may tend to avoid people who you consider are likely to criticize you or you may criticize others before they criticize you. You may also play safe and avoid taking risks that may lead to you being criticized. Thus, fear of criticism tends to promote conformity and inhibits creative and innovative thinking which if expressed to others may attract criticism.

Not being accepted, liked or loved by significant others

If you depreciate yourself when you think that another person either does not accept you, does not like you or does not love you, then you tend to think of yourself as unacceptable, unlikeable or unlovable. If you are particularly prone to self-depreciation in the face of these conditions then you tend to infer that another does not accept you, for example, in the absence of evidence that this is the case. Or if another person does show that they dislike you and you put yourself down, then you overestimate the number of other people who may also dislike you.

When you put yourself down for being disliked, for example, since you also believe that you need to be liked you will go out of your way to be liked by the person who dislikes you. Thus, you may sacrifice your own interests in order to get back into the good books of the person who dislikes you, which you probably wouldn't do if you did not depreciate yourself about being disliked. If you are particularly prone to depreciating yourself for not being accepted, liked or loved, then you will do all you can to be accepted before there is any hint of a threat that the other person may dislike you. Thus, you may attempt to ingratiate yourself with others you have just met, a tactic which sometimes backfires because some people will dislike you for your ingratiating behaviour whereas they would have liked you if you were more genuine with them.

Having a defect or handicap

When you depreciate yourself for having some kind of defect or handicap, you again begin by rating the defect or handicap negatively and then overgeneralize by rating your self negatively. You can put yourself down for a range of defects or handicaps, examples being obesity, stammering and dyslexia.

When you depreciate yourself for having a defect or a handicap, you are doing two things. First, you are labelling something about you as a defect or a handicap, and second, you depreciate yourself for having the defect or disability. Not everybody regards being obese as a defect, for example, and even among those who do, not everyone depreciates themselves for having this condition.

The role of others is important here, but it is complex. I would say that the more others regard something about you as a defect or a handicap, the more likely it is that you will regard this aspect in the same way and the more likely it is that you will depreciate yourself. However, this is not always the case, as is demonstrated in a condition known as Body Dysmorphic Disorder (BDD). In BDD (which is often referred to as perceived ugliness syndrome in the media), the person thinks that some aspect of her appearance is very ugly and she depreciates herself for being defective in this way. The point, however, is that other people do not think that the person has a defect. This makes little or no difference to the person with BDD, who will not accept evidence that this is the case. The important point is not what others actually think, but what the person thinks about herself, which she then projects on to others. As one of my BDD clients once said: 'Since I know that I am a hideous person for having a large nose, I am convinced that others think of me in the same way, and even when they say they do not, they are lying to me.'

If you depreciate yourself for having a defect or handicap, you then overestimate the extent to which others regard that aspect as a defect or handicap and think badly about you as a result. You also experience a strong tendency to avoid situations where your defect or handicap will become apparent to others. Since you overestimate the extent to which your defect or handicap is apparent to others, your avoidant behaviour is likely to be widespread.

The impact of self-depreciation on your relationships

As you will have seen from what I have already discussed, if you depreciate yourself, this process can have a negative impact on your relationships with other people. The way you relate to other people when you depreciate yourself is affected quite a lot by how you view these other people when you are in a self-depreciating state of mind. These views of other people and how you act towards them can take a number of different forms, and I will briefly outline two to show you how problematic your relationships can be when you put yourself down.

1 When you see yourself as an incompetent person, you may tend to see others as competent and in your dealings with them you will not expect that they will be interested in what you have to say. You may also take their opinions as facts, thus disregarding your own. Consequently, you easily comply with their wishes and can be easily moulded by them if they are manipulative. In more extreme cases, you may put those whom you see as especially competent on a pedestal and think that they would not be interested in you at all. Thus, when you meet them you are very deferential and become embarrassed in their presence.

2 If you base your worth as a person on being approved then you will tend to see yourself as unlikeable if someone who is significant to you does not approve of you. You will tend to think that the other person has more worth than you and you will try anything to get into his good books. This means that you will tend to be compliant and unassertive in your dealings with him. You will tend to go out of your way to please him, again tending to subjugate your own desires in deference to his wishes. Even when you do manage to gain the other person's approval, you act anxiously around him in case you do something which leads him to think poorly of you. If the person claims to like you, you will still not relax and show the real you because you think that he only likes you because of the facade that you have constructed and that if he truly got to know you he couldn't possibly like you. Thus, if you think of yourself as unlikeable then you will find it difficult to be genuine in your relationships with those whose approval you think you need.

Views of the self in self-depreciation

When you depreciate yourself, you can put yourself down in various ways. In this section I will briefly list these different views of yourself. Please note that all of these different forms of self-depreciation involve you evaluating your self in a global, negative and pejorative way. I will discuss this further in the next chapter.

8

'I am bad' – here you judge your self negatively in the moral sphere. This form of self-judgment is most often found in guilt.

'I am worthless' – here you judge your self as having no value to you as well as to others. This form of self-judgment is most often found in depression and anxiety.

'I am unlikeable/unlovable' – here you judge your self in terms of your lack of appeal to others. This form of self-judgment is found in a number of emotional problems, including depression, anxiety, hurt and unhealthy jealousy.

'I am insignificant' – here you regard yourself as having little or no importance, whereas others are seen as having much more importance. This form of self-judgment is most often seen in shame and lack of self-assertion.

'I am defective' – here you consider that there is something radically wrong with your self. This form of self-judgment is most often found in shame.

'I am repulsive' – here you consider that you are hideous to yourself and others and this often relates to an important aspect of your appearance. This form of self-judgment is again most often found in shame.

'I am useless' – here you regard yourself as having no utilitarian value to the world. This form of self-judgment is most often found in depression.

'I am stupid' – here you tend to judge yourself on the basis of your incompetence or self-defeating behaviour. This form of self-judgment is most often found in unhealthy anger towards yourself.

'I am inferior' – here you judge your self in relation to others and are found wanting in that comparison. This form of self-judgment is most often found in unhealthy envy, shame, anxiety and depression.

'I am pathetic' – here you rate yourself for having an unacceptable weakness or for acting weakly. This type of self-judgment is particularly found in shame and unhealthy anger towards yourself.

While I have discussed stark forms of self-depreciation, I should also make clear that self-depreciation may take more subtle forms. For example, while you may not consider yourself to be worthless for failing to achieve a valued goal, you still may consider yourself to be less worthy for failing in this respect than you would be if you succeeded. This is an example of what Howard Young, a noted REBT (Rational Emotive Behaviour Therapy) therapist (sadly deceased), used to call 'less me' thinking. Deservingness is also a subtle form of self-depreciation, as in the situation where you have failed and believe that you are undeserving of good fortune as a result. I am not talking here about a situation where failure on its own precludes reward (e.g. you fail an exam and are not awarded a degree), but about being denied a reward because you as a person do not deserve one.

Having outlined some of the major forms of self-depreciation, let me conclude this chapter by discussing three important distinctions with respect to self-depreciation: general versus specific self-depreciation, conditional versus unconditional self-depreciation and explicit versus implicit self-depreciation.

Specific and general self-depreciation

Virtually all, if not all, humans depreciate themselves in some area of their lives – even those who write books on how to develop self-acceptance! Thus, the complete eradication of self-depreciation is an unrealistic human goal. However, some people depreciate themselves in many areas of their lives (and can thus be said to experience general self-depreciation) whereas others only do so in specific areas. While this book is written for both groups of people, it is important that you appreciate that it will take longer to develop self-acceptance when you experience general self-depreciation. Having said this, if you only put yourself down in one or two situations in life, doing so can limit your life considerably if these situations are central to your life and if you have a chronic longstanding problem in this specific area. Even if you experience general self-depreciation it is important to begin to address this general problem by tackling specific examples, as I shall discuss further in Chapter 9.

The purpose of this book is to equip you with the knowledge and skills that you will need to begin the journey towards self-acceptance. If you implement this knowledge and these skills in the longer term, you will become more self-accepting both in general terms and in specific situations where you currently depreciate yourself. This process will be longer if you experience general rather than specific self-depreciation, because in the former you put yourself down in a much broader set of circumstances than in the latter. However, if you are persistent and patient then your efforts will pay off.

A word of caution, however. No matter how much effort you put into implementing the knowledge and techniques that I describe in this book, you will still depreciate yourself under certain conditions. Why? Because it is not within the capacity of human beings to reach and sustain perfect levels of complete and utter self-acceptance, which once attained are never lost. No, the best that you can strive for is greater and greater self-acceptance, which in itself will improve your mental well-being tremendously.

Conditional and unconditional self-depreciation

In most cases, your self-depreciation is likely to be conditional. This means that you tend to depreciate yourself when certain conditions exist. For example, you think of yourself as a failure when you fail at an important task. However, if you had succeeded at this task then you would not have depreciated yourself. This is not to say that you would necessarily regard yourself as *a success* (although of course you could). It is just that, in this case, failure triggers your self-depreciation, whereas success does not. In this sense, your self-depreciation is conditional upon you failing. The following is a list of other examples of conditional self-depreciation. The statement in brackets spells out the conditionality of the self-depreciation.

'I am unworthy if I get rejected (but if I am accepted I do not think of myself as unworthy).'

'I am bad when I break my moral code (but when I live up to this code I am not a bad person).'

'I am unlovable when someone I care for is angry with me (but when they are nice to me, I am not unlovable).'

'I am a disgusting person because I am so unattractive (but I would not be a disgusting person if I were attractive).'

Conditional forms of self-depreciation are also apparent in what Howard Young called 'less me' thinking. Consider the following:

'I am less worthy if I fail my exam than if I pass it.'

'I would be more likeable if my new flatmate liked me than if she didn't.'

'I would be a better person if I helped my parents than if I didn't.'

When self-depreciation is unconditional your negative evaluation of yourself does not change with changing conditions. Let me take the above examples and demonstrate the unconditional versions of these conditional self-depreciation statements.

'I am unworthy if I get rejected (even if I am accepted I am still unworthy).'

'I am bad when I break my moral code (and even if I live up to this code I am still a bad person).'

'I am unlovable when someone I care for is angry with me (and even if they are nice to me, I am still unlovable).'

'I am a disgusting person because I am so unattractive (even if I were attractive, I would still be disgusting).'

'I am unworthy whether or not I fail my exam.'

'I am unlikeable whether or not my new flatmate likes me.'

'I am a bad person whether I help my parents or not.'

In unconditional self-depreciation, then, you consider yourself to be bad, unworthy or defective, for example, and you can think of no conditions that can rescue you from this psychological state. Indeed, if you depreciate yourself unconditionally, you do not regard this as a psychological state. Rather, you regard it as a fact. Unconditional self-depreciation, then, is more serious than conditional self-depreciation. If your self-depreciation is unconditional, you may still derive benefit from reading this book and from the exercises that I will describe presently. However, you probably need to see a counsellor or therapist to address this issue more fully. Thus, if you recognize that your self-depreciation is unconditional, I suggest that you discuss this in the first instance with your doctor, who will suggest an appropriate referral.

Explicit and implicit self-depreciation

The final issue that I want to discuss concerns whether your self-depreciation is explicit or implicit. When you put yourself down, you can do so either explicitly or implicitly. When your self-depreciation is explicit it is clearly stated in what you say about yourself (e.g. 'If I failed my exam I would be unworthy') or it is clearly present in your thinking about yourself. However, when your self-depreciation is implicit, it is present, but not stated in either what you say about yourself or how you think of yourself. For example, you may say or think explicitly: 'If I failed my exam, I would really muck things up for myself' and mean just that and only that, in which case you would not be putting yourself down. On the other hand, you may say or think explicitly: 'If I failed my exam, I would really muck things up for myself' and really mean implicitly: 'If I failed my exam, I would be unworthy.' For all sorts of reasons you may not want to admit to yourself that you really mean the latter, so you hide this realization from yourself.

A common form of implicit self-depreciation occurs in what on the surface is stated as trait or appearance descriptions of yourself (e.g. 'I am shy' or 'I am fat'), in negative evaluations of a role that you occupy (e.g. 'I am a bad mother') or in negative evaluations of performance (e.g. 'I really gave a bad presentation'). When self-depreciation is implicit in these statements you really mean the following: 'I am shy (and therefore inadequate)', 'I am fat (and therefore disgusting)', 'I am a bad mother (and therefore a bad person)', 'I really gave a bad presentation (and am therefore less worthy than I would be if I gave a good presentation)'.

However, the same statement might not involve self-depreciation. Thus, you may describe yourself as shy and accept yourself for it even though you might wish you were more confident socially, which you might wish to pursue as a goal. Similarly, you may describe yourself as fat and accept yourself for it. If you didn't like your fatness you might seek assistance to lose weight or, equally, you may like being fat.

How you can tell if you are depreciating yourself

Explicit statements are not always a good guide to self-depreciation, so how can you tell if you are depreciating yourself? There are four ways: by inspecting your emotions; by identifying what you really believe; by examining the way you act or 'feel like' acting; and by considering the ways in which you subsequently think. Let me consider each one in turn.

1 *Inspect your emotions.* Self-depreciation tends to lead to unhealthy negative emotions about negative life events, whereas self-acceptance tends to lead to healthy negative emotions about those same events. So if you experience anxiety, depression, guilt, shame, unhealthy jealousy, ego-defensive anger, hurt or unhealthy envy and your attitude towards yourself is the point at issue, then it is likely that you are putting yourself

down, whereas if you experience concern, sadness, remorse, disappointment, healthy jealousy, healthy anger, regret and healthy envy, it is likely that you are not depreciating yourself.

2 *Identify what you really believe.* If you are unsure whether or not you are depreciating yourself, ask yourself what you really believe in the situation in question. Don't just inspect your surface thoughts about the event in question, focus on what you really believe. Your feelings will also help in this respect. Indeed, if you truly believe that you are inadequate for falling far short of your ideal in a given situation AND you feel ashamed in this situation, then there is a very good chance that you were depreciating yourself in this episode.

3 *Examine your actions and your action tendencies.* When you put yourself down this has a great bearing on the way you act or 'feel like' acting (or what are known as action tendencies). Self-depreciation tends to lead to actions that are self-defeating or potentially self-defeating (in the case of action tendencies), whereas self-acceptance tends to lead to actions that are constructive or potentially constructive (in the case of action tendencies).

4 *Consider the ways in which you subsequently think.* When you put yourself down the thinking that you subsequently engage in is unrealistic and biased, whereas when you accept yourself your subsequent thinking tends to be realistic and balanced.

When self-depreciation isn't self-depreciation

Psychologists distinguish between words and their meaning. Thus, sometimes when you use the language of self-depreciation you are not, in fact, putting yourself down. When Michael accidentally broke an expensive vase he exclaimed, 'I am such an idiot.' However, he did not feel angry with himself (anger at self would be a sign that he was condemning himself); rather he felt annoyed at his clumsiness (which indicated that he was not putting himself down).

In addition, by their language, some people seem to put themselves down, but in reality they are feigning self-depreciation to ward off criticism from others and/or to get what they want from them. Thus, Michele procrastinated on her essay and went to see her tutor to ask for an extension. Her tutor was well known for being tough with students who were late with their work and rarely granted extensions. When she was in his room,

Michele tearfully confessed the fact that she hadn't completed her work and expressed the view that she was a failure for not handing her essay in on time. Her tutor responded with sympathy and understanding, and told her that she was not a failure and that these things sometimes happen. To Michele's secret and concealed satisfaction, her tutor gave her a week's extension. As soon as she left his room, Michele smiled ruefully and that night she boasted to her friends how she feigned tears to get what she wanted from her tutor.

In this chapter, I have considered the different forms that self-depreciation takes and have shown how putting yourself down affects the way you feel, act and subsequently think. It is not easy tackling self-depreciation and working towards acquiring the healthy attitude of self-acceptance, but it can be done if you are prepared to work at it. The first step in acquiring a healthier attitude towards yourself is to understand the concept of self-acceptance and to appreciate why it is more effective in promoting psychological health in the longer term than the concept of self-esteem. This is the subject of the following chapter.

2

The Importance of Unconditional Self-acceptance

The chances are that, if you are reading this book, you tend to put yourself down either in specific situations or more generally. If the latter is the case, you would probably say that you suffer from low self-esteem. It may be that you are hoping that reading this book will help to raise your self-esteem. If so, I am not going to help you to do this. No, your eyes have not deceived you. I am not going to help you to raise or improve your self-esteem. Why not? Because self-esteem is not a useful concept and if you begin to like yourself more this has its problems. You are probably confused about what I've just written, but trust me – all will become clear presently. Let me begin my explanation about why improving your self-esteem will not help you in the long term by defining what we mean by self-esteem.

What is self-esteem?

In order for you to understand what self-esteem is, I first have to define the terms 'self' and 'esteem'. Let's begin with the term 'self'. What is the self? Let me see if I can help you to answer this question by asking you a further set of questions.

- Are your actions or behaviour part of your self?
- Are your thoughts part of your self?
- Are your personality characteristics part of your self?
- Are your feelings and emotions part of your self?
- Are your sensations part of your self?
- Are your images or pictures that you see in your mind's eye part of your self?
- Are your dreams part of your self?
- Are your bodily parts part of your self?

In all probability you have answered 'yes' to all eight questions because you realize that all these different aspects are either a part of you, authored by you or experienced by you. My colleague Paul Hauck has provided a very useful definition of the self. He says that the self is 'every conceivable thing about you that can be rated'. All of the aspects that I asked you about in the above eight questions can be rated and thus form a part of your self.

16

Taking this approach, your self, then, is extraordinarily complex since it encompasses all the behaviour you have performed in your life, all the thoughts, images and dreams you have had, all the feelings and sensations you have experienced, and so on. Also, it is important to note that the self is a process and changes over time. Your self today, therefore, is not exactly the same as it was yesterday, nor will it be the same tomorrow.

So what is not a part of your self? Well, your possessions are not part of your self. You may object here and cite your most prized possession which has great importance to you. However, I would say that it is your feelings about this possession which are part of your self and not the possession itself, which exists as an entity independent of you. It is the independent existence of an object or person that makes it not a part of your self, no matter how important that object or person is to you and no matter how much you 'feel' they are a part of your self.

Let me present a diagrammatic summary of what I have said so far about the self.

Self

The self is every conceivable thing about you that can be rated:

- behaviour
- thoughts
- personality characteristics
- feelings and emotions
- sensations
- images
- dreams
- bodily parts.

The self is extremely complex.
The self is constantly changing.

Now let's consider the term 'esteem'. It comes from the verb 'to estimate', which means to judge, rate or evaluate. So what does self-esteem mean? It means rating the self.

Now here is the problem. Can you legitimately give your self a rating or evaluation that can do full justice to it, given that, as we have already seen, the self is exceedingly complex and constantly changing? The answer is a resounding NO. Thus, if you have low self-esteem you are consistently giving your exceedingly complex and changing self a single, global, negative rating. The remedy is not to give your exceedingly complex and changing self a global positive rating, which is what you would have to do if you wanted high self-esteem. So if improving your self-esteem is not the alternative to self-depreciation, what is? The answer is developing unconditional self-acceptance.

What is unconditional self-acceptance (USA)?

The concept of unconditional self-acceptance (USA) is best explained by considering a set of principles which I will discuss one at a time. In doing so, I will outline where applicable the relevant principle underlying self-depreciation.

1 As a human being you cannot legitimately be given a single rating, but parts of you can be rated, as can what happens to you

I have already made the point that human beings are incredibly complex. Thus, you are a complex mix of behaviours, thoughts, personality characteristics, feelings and emotions, sensations, images, dreams and bodily parts. How on earth are you going to arrive at a legitimate single rating that completely accounts for you in all your complexity? The answer is that you can't do this. Also, even if you could give yourself a single rating, this would soon be out of date because as soon as you assigned a rating to yourself, you would have moved on, acquiring more experience and processing them in slightly new ways. In short, it is not possible to assign a process like your self a rating, which is by definition a fixed thing.

You can, however, rate parts of yourself and the events in your life and it is important that you do so, otherwise you will not be motivated to change negative aspects of your self and negative life events.

When you depreciate yourself you are operating under a very different principle. This principle states that human beings can be given a single global rating. Thus, when you believe that you are inadequate, you are assigning to yourself a single, negative, global rating (i.e. inadequate) which is unwarranted.

2 As a human being your essence is that you are fallible and unique

Can we say that as human beings we have an essence, a feature that all humans share, that defines us? In my view our essence is twofold. First, all humans are fallible. We all make mistakes. As my colleague Dr Maxie C. Maultsby Jr has said, all humans have an incurable error-making tendency. Your second essential feature is summed up in the song title 'There'll never be another you'. In other words, you are unique. Even if we cloned you, you and your clone would not be identical since you would each have different experiences. To sum up: if you have an essence as a human it is that you are fallible and unique.

When you depreciate yourself you are operating under a very different principle, namely, human beings are perfectible. Thus, when you fail to achieve your standards and depreciate yourself you tend to do so because you believe that once you set goals for yourself, you must, literally must, achieve these goals.

3 You are equal to other humans in terms of shared humanity, but unequal in many specific respects

If you cannot legitimately rate another person, then it follows that one person is not worthier than another, for assigning worth to a person is a form of rating a person. Rather, it makes more sense and is more accurate to say that all humans are equal in being human but unequal in many different respects. Thus, I may be better at practising psychology than you, but you may be better at gardening than me. I may be more persistent at doing tasks than you, but you may be more creative at these tasks than me.

It follows from this that it is not realistic or helpful for you to compare your self with the self of another person, but it is realistic and helpful for you to compare your behaviour or any other rateable aspect with that of another person. This aspect-based comparison can help you to learn from others who are better than you at the aspect under consideration, whereas self-based comparison can only lead you to feelings of superiority or, more often, feelings of inferiority.

When you depreciate yourself you do think that selves can be compared and that human beings differ in worth. When you come off worse in such comparisons, you render yourself very vulnerable to depression, anxiety and other emotional disorders.

4 When you accept yourself unconditionally, you think logically and avoid overgeneralization errors

When you depreciate yourself you tend to make illogical overgeneralizations. In particular, you make what is known as the part–whole error. In this error you focus on and rate a part of yourself and then on the basis of this rating you rate your whole self. For example, Maurice gave a presentation at work and because he was so nervous he kept putting on the wrong overheads. After the presentation, Maurice felt ashamed because he thought that he gave a poor performance at the presentation and, more crucially, because he thought that he was a defective person for his poor performance. Maurice's part–whole error is revealed in the following: because I gave a poor presentation (part), therefore I am a defective person (whole).

In counselling, I helped Maurice to see that while he may have given a poor performance at the presentation, this only proved that he was a fallible human being who was capable of doing well and poorly, and that he was not a defective person. Maurice then refrained from rating his self (whole) on the basis of his performance at the presentation (part) and thus was no longer guilty of making the part–whole error.

5 Unconditional self-acceptance is closely linked with a flexible, preferential philosophy

The ideas in this book are based on a therapeutic approach known as Rational Emotive Behaviour Therapy (REBT) which was originated in the mid-1950s by an American clinical psychologist called Albert Ellis. Ellis noted early on that people's self-depreciation was closely linked with their tendency to make absolute demands on themselves. For instance, Albert Ellis would show Maurice in the above example that the reason he was depreciating himself as a defective person was because he was demanding that he must give a good performance at his presentation and he didn't do so. Ellis later argued that frequently self-depreciation stems from a demand about the self (and sometimes about others) which has not been met. However, other REBT therapists argue that self-depreciation and demands about self and others which are not met are linked, and do not argue that self-depreciation stems from unmet demands. Sometimes, these therapists argue, demands about self stem from self-depreciation. Whichever is the case, for our purposes here, if you want to develop unconditional self-acceptance, it is important that you challenge both self-depreciation beliefs and demands about self (and sometimes about others).

If self-depreciation beliefs are closely linked to demands about self and others, what are self-acceptance beliefs linked to? The answer is 'full preferences' about self and others. Full preferences take the form of wishes, wants, desires and the like, but they also state that one does not have to get what one wishes, wants or desires. When these full preference beliefs cluster together to make a philosophy this is called a flexible, preferential philosophy, which contrasts markedly with the rigid, demanding philosophy that is closely linked with self-depreciation.

Let me suggest an exercise to help you determine whether or not you have grasped this point. I am going to list some demands and full preferences (in List 1) and then some self-depreciation and self-acceptance beliefs (in List 2). Your task is to determine which beliefs from each list go together.

List 1

1 I want people to like me, but they don't have to.
2 I absolutely must do well at my job.
3 I absolutely should not have hurt my mother's feelings.

4 People must like me.
5 I don't want to reveal any weaknesses in public, but there is no reason why I must not do this.
6 I want to do well at my job, but I don't absolutely have to do so.
7 I must not reveal any weaknesses in public.
8 I wish I hadn't hurt my mother's feelings, but there is no reason which suggests that I am immune from doing so.
9 I must be more attractive than I am.
10 I'd like to be more attractive than I am, but it isn't essential that I be so.

List 2

1 I am a bad person for hurting my mother's feelings.
2 I am not worthless for being unattractive. I am acceptable because I am alive, unique and human.
3 I am defective if I reveal a weakness in public.
4 I am not a bad person for hurting my mother's feelings. I am a regular person who acted badly.
5 If people do not like me, it proves that I am unlikeable.
6 If I reveal a weakness in public it does not mean that I am defective. It means that I am an ordinary human being with strengths and weaknesses.
7 If people do not like me it does not mean that I am unlikeable. It means that I am a fallible human being with some likeable and unlikeable aspects whom some people will like and others won't.
8 If I don't do well at my job it proves that I am a failure.
9 If I don't do well at my job it does not mean that I am a failure. It means that I am an unrateable fallible human being who has not done well in this area of life at this time.
10 I am worthless for being unattractive.

How many did you get right? The correct answers are as follows:

List 1	List 2
1	7
2	8
3	1
4	5

5	6
6	9
7	3
8	4
9	10
10	2

Here is a list of how the relevant full preferences and self-acceptance beliefs, on the one hand, and the relevant demands and self-depreciation beliefs, on the other hand, go together.

- I want people to like me, but they don't have to. If people do not like me it does not mean that I am unlikeable. It means that I am a fallible human being with some likeable and unlikeable aspects whom some people will like and others won't.
- People must like me. If people do not like me, it proves that I am unlikeable.

- I want to do well at my job, but I don't absolutely have to do so. If I don't do well at my job it does not mean that I am a failure. It means that I am an unrateable fallible human being who has not done well in this area of life at this time.
- I absolutely must do well at my job. If I don't do well at my job it proves that I am a failure.

- I wish I hadn't hurt my mother's feelings, but there is no reason which suggests that I am immune from doing so. I am not a bad person for hurting my mother's feelings. I am a regular person who acted badly.
- I absolutely should not have hurt my mother's feelings. I am a bad person for doing so.

- I don't want to reveal any weaknesses in public, but there is no reason why I must not do this. If I do reveal a weakness in public it does not mean that I am defective. It means that I am an ordinary human being with strengths and weaknesses.

- I must not reveal any weaknesses in public and I am defective if I do so.

- I'd like to be more attractive than I am, but it isn't essential that I be so. I am not worthless for being unattractive. I am acceptable because I am alive, unique and human.
- I must be more attractive than I am. I am worthless for being unattractive.

Now that I have explained the connection between self-acceptance beliefs and full preferences and that between self-depreciation beliefs and demands, I will proceed to the sixth principle of self-acceptance.

6 When you accept yourself unconditionally, your emotions are healthy and your behaviour is constructive

In Chapter 1, I showed how self-depreciation is involved in a range of emotional and behavioural problems. Thus, when you depreciate yourself in the face of a negative activating event you tend to experience one or more unhealthy negative emotions such as anxiety, depression, guilt, hurt, shame, unhealthy anger, unhealthy jealousy and unhealthy envy. However, when you accept yourself in the face of the same negative activating event you tend to experience one or more healthy negative emotions such as concern, sadness, remorse, regret, disappointment, healthy anger, healthy jealousy and healthy envy. The following is a set of representative self-depreciating beliefs and their emotional effects and a corresponding set of self-acceptance beliefs and their different emotional effects. For clarity, I will first consider the unhealthy emotion and its self-depreciating belief before presenting its healthy alternative based on self-acceptance.

Anxiety:	'If I fail at my upcoming test which I must not do, I will be a failure.'
Concern:	'I would rather not fail at my upcoming test, but there is no law of the universe to prevent me from doing so. If I do fail, I will not be a failure. Rather I will be a fallible human being who has failed.'
Depression:	'Since my partner rejected me, as she absolutely should not have done, this means that I am no good.'
Sadness:	'I would have preferred it had my partner not rejected me, but there is no reason why she absolutely should not have done so. Even though she rejected me, I am still a fallible human being. There is no evidence that I am no good.'

23

Guilt: 'I have hurt the feelings of my parents, which I absolutely should not have done. I am therefore a bad person.'

Remorse: 'I have hurt the feelings of my parents. I would rather not have done so, but there is no reason why I absolutely should not have done so. I am a fallible human being for doing the wrong thing rather than a bad person.'

Hurt: 'My ex-girlfriend is going out with my best friend, which absolutely should not happen. Since it is happening, this proves that I am unlovable.'

Sorrow: 'My ex-girlfriend is going out with my best friend. I would much rather that she did not do this, but I don't have to get this desire met. The fact that she is going out with him has no bearing on the way I view my whole self. I am fallible rather than unlovable.'

Shame: 'I have acted foolishly in front of my peers which I absolutely should not have done, and this proves that I am an inadequate person.'

Disappointment: 'I have acted foolishly in front of my peers. There is no reason why I absolutely should not have done so even though I would have preferred it if I hadn't. I am not an inadequate person for acting in the way that I did. Rather, I am a complex, unrateable human being.'

Unhealthy anger: 'You absolutely should not have criticized me. Your criticism reminds me that I am a failure.'

Healthy anger: 'I would rather you hadn't criticized me, but there's no reason why you absolutely should not have done so. Your criticism reminds me that I am fallible and not a failure.'

Unhealthy jealousy: 'If my husband looks at another woman, which he must not do, it means that he finds her more attractive than me. This must not happen, but if it does it proves that I am worthless.'

Healthy jealousy: 'I would prefer it if my husband does not look at another woman or does not find her more attractive than me. However, there is no law forbidding him from doing either. If he does, I can still accept myself as a fallible human being who is equal in humanity with everyone else. It does not prove that I am worthless.'

Unhealthy envy: 'My friend is making more money at his job than I am. I must have what he has and because I don't this makes me less worthy than I would be if I had what he has.'

Healthy envy: 'My friend is making more money at his job than I am. I would prefer it if I was making as much as him, but I do not have to do so. I am not less worthy than I would be if I earned as much as my friend. Rather, I am the same fallible, unrateable human whether I have what he has or not.'

In addition, if you hold a self-acceptance belief you are more likely to act in constructive ways, whereas when you hold a corresponding self-depreciation belief you tend to act in self-defeating ways. For example, if you believe you are a failure for doing poorly at a task at work, you will tend to stop working at the task and turn away from searching for ways in which you can learn from your errors. You will be hesitant in doing similar tasks in the future, avoiding them whenever you can. However, if you accept yourself as an ordinary human with your successes and failures rather than as a failure, you are more likely to keep working at the task and will actively search for ways of learning from your mistakes. You will be somewhat wary of attempting similar tasks, but you will still do so.

7 *If you still want to rate yourself, judge yourself against conditions that do not change in your lifetime, think of yourself as worthwhile because you are human, alive, unique and constantly changing*

As I have already shown, one of the main features of self-depreciation is the rating that you make of your self. I have argued earlier that rating your self is illegitimate in that you are too complex to merit such a judgment, and in any case you are not a static entity, but an organism constantly in flux. The alternative, then, to rating the self is to acknowledge that you are human, alive, fallible and unique whatever you do, and to accept yourself for being so. However, you may be among those who still want to rate themselves. You want to regard yourself as a worthy person or a good person, for example. Is there a way of doing this without being vulnerable to emotional disturbance? Yes, there is. You can choose to rate yourself as a worthwhile person as long as you do so unconditionally. This position is known as unconditional high self-esteem. It means that you base your worth on conditions that do not change. What are these conditions? The fact that as long as you are alive you are human, fallible, unique and changing. Thus, there is very little chance that you will wake up one day transformed into an animal, become infallible, be an exact replica of someone else and stop changing. So as long as you believe that you are worthwhile because you are alive, human, fallible, unique and changing, then you will not experience emotional disturbance, at least in relation to your feelings about yourself.

Of course you can't prove that you are worthwhile in the same way that you can prove that you are alive, human, fallible, unique and constantly changing, so you are making a leap of faith. Someone could come up with the equally valid view that you are worthless because you are alive, human, fallible, unique and constantly changing. But if you are going to rate yourself this is probably the safest way of doing so.

There are other ways of rating yourself that are conditional which do not have to lead to emotional disturbance. Thus, if you believe that you are worthwhile because Jesus loves you or that you have a fairy godmother looking after you, as long as you believe this you will be fine. But the trouble is that one day you may think that Jesus hates you or you may stop believing in the existence of fairy godmothers, and then you will become vulnerable to emotional disturbance (e.g. I am worthless because Jesus hates me).

In short, the safest of all solutions to the problem of self-depreciation is unconditional self-acceptance where you do not rate yourself at all. But if you want to rate yourself, then unconditional high self-esteem is far better than all forms of conditional self-esteem, which are at the core of self-depreciation.

8 Unconditional self-acceptance promotes constructive action, not resignation

Unfortunately, the word 'acceptance' conjures up resignation in some people's minds. If you think this, you may well believe that accepting yourself means resigning yourself to the fact that there is nothing you can do to change aspects of yourself that you don't like and that are self-defeating. However, the good news is that the opposite is true. When you depreciate yourself you label your self with the behaviour that you wish to change. If you act selfishly, you are a selfish (and therefore a bad) person. If you act foolishly, you are a fool (and therefore unworthy). Labelling yourself increases, rather than decreases, the chances that you will resign yourself to repeating self-defeating patterns of behaviour. It is as if you are saying to yourself: 'Since I am a fool, how can I learn to act non-foolishly? The answer is, I can't.'

However, unconditional self-acceptance means viewing yourself in a much more complex and flexible way. You see yourself as someone who can and does act selfishly and non-selfishly, as someone who can act foolishly and sensibly. Since you do not label yourself with your behaviour when you accept yourself unconditionally, you are much more likely to see that change is possible than when you depreciate yourself.

In short, when you accept yourself unconditionally for acting negatively, for example, you do the following:

- You acknowledge that you have behaved negatively.
- You regret acting in the way that you did.
- You acknowledge that regrettably all the conditions were in place for you to act in the way that you did.
- You recognize that you can learn from this experience.
- You review all the relevant factors that were involved in leading you to behave negatively.
- You decide what you can do differently in future.
- You commit yourself to act differently in future.

I hope you can see from the foregoing that rather than encouraging resignation, unconditional self-acceptance promotes constructive change.

9 You can learn to accept yourself unconditionally (but never perfectly, nor for all time)

This ninth principle states that unconditional self-acceptance is a way of thinking that can be learned. If it wasn't, I would not have bothered to write this book, nor would I run courses on helping people to develop unconditional self-acceptance. However, it is also true that in all probability you will not be able to apply this philosophy perfectly so that you never depreciate yourself again. It is against the principle of human fallibility for you to do anything perfectly over time, and developing perfect, once-and-for-all-time self-acceptance is therefore almost impossible for any human. The best that you can hope for is to work towards ever greater self-acceptance and accept the grim reality that, even if you rigorously practise the principles and techniques that I outline in this book, you will, at times, still depreciate yourself. This is a realistic position, and only those of you who are looking for perfect self-acceptance are likely to be discouraged by it.

10 Internalizing unconditional self-acceptance is difficult and involves hard work

Wouldn't it be great if internalizing unconditional self-acceptance was easy and all you had to do was to read this book – not act on it, just read it? Yes, it would be great, but as you can probably tell from my tone, it isn't that easy. Indeed, it isn't easy at all. Developing unconditional self-acceptance involves a lot of persistent practice in challenging unhealthy demands and self-depreciation beliefs and acting in ways that are consistent with the healthy alternatives to these beliefs. Indeed, the more ingrained your self-depreciation beliefs, the harder you will have to work to uproot them and replace them with self-accepting beliefs. The same is true with self-depreciation beliefs that are general (rather than specific) and unconditional (rather than conditional) – see pp. 10–11 for a discussion of specific versus general self-depreciation and pp. 11–12 for a discussion of conditional verses unconditional self-depreciation.

The more you accept the grim reality that developing unconditional self-acceptance is difficult, the more you will put into practice what you learn from this book. Thus, if you are looking for an easy solution to your self-depreciation problems, sadly you will not find it here.

11 Internalizing unconditional self-acceptance requires force and energy

The final principle of unconditional self-acceptance states that if you really want to internalize this philosophy (as much as you humanly can), then you need to do so forcefully and with energy. If you try to adopt a self-accepting philosophy in a weak, half-hearted, 'namby-pamby' manner, then it just won't take. Why? Because you probably hold your self-depreciating beliefs with a strong degree of conviction and therefore challenging these strongly held views with weak insipid methods just won't work. To achieve psychological change you often have to fight fire with fire, so if you want to change your strongly held self-depreciating ideas you do have to do so with strength, force and energy.

In summary, I present the eleven principles of unconditional self-acceptance below. Why not take a copy of it and read it several times a day to remind yourself what unconditional self-acceptance means?

1 As a human being you cannot legitimately be given a single rating, but parts of you can be rated, as can what happens to you.
2 As a human being your essence is that you are fallible and unique.
3 You are equal to other humans in terms of shared humanity, but unequal in many specific respects.

4 When you accept yourself unconditionally, you think logically and avoid overgeneralization errors.

5 Unconditional self-acceptance is closely linked with a flexible, preferential philosophy.

6 When you accept yourself unconditionally, your emotions are healthy and your behaviour is constructive.

7 If you still want to rate yourself, judge yourself against conditions that do not change in your lifetime. Thus, think of yourself as worthwhile because you are human, alive, unique and constantly changing.

8 Unconditional self-acceptance promotes constructive action, not resignation.

9 You can learn to accept yourself unconditionally (but never perfectly, nor for all time).

10 Internalizing unconditional self-acceptance is difficult and involves hard work.

11 Internalizing unconditional self-acceptance requires force and energy.

3

Specify Your Problems and Set Goals

The first step in any self-change programme is to be clear with yourself what your problems are and to set goals in relation to these problems. It is important, therefore, to know where you are and where you are going. Since this is a book on dealing with problems which involve you putting yourself down in some way, for the purpose of getting the most out of what follows specify your self-depreciation problems and choose goals which involve you achieving some measure of unconditional self-acceptance. To help you with this and with the other methods that I will introduce in the subsequent chapters, I will present the case of someone I helped to become more self-accepting. The person, who I will call Mandy, was a client of mine who went through the same self-acceptance programme that I describe in this book but did so in individual counselling.

Before I begin, let me be clear about what I can help you to achieve in this book and what I can't help you to achieve. The best way of viewing this book and its contents is to regard it as a manual, the purpose of which is to help you to take the initial steps along the difficult path towards self-acceptance. I will be presenting and discussing a number of techniques for you to use on your own. I will describe them in detail and alert you to common difficulties that people have experienced in putting them into practice. I will also discuss what you can do to surmount these difficulties. So, I can equip you with the major tools that you will need in your journey towards greater self-acceptance. What I cannot do is to help you achieve the state of full unconditional self-acceptance. Self-acceptance is as process rather than a static entity. What I can say is that if you commit yourself to applying the methods described in this book regularly over time, then in all probability you will make great strides along the path towards self-acceptance. If you just read the book without doing any of the exercises described herein, you will have a good read and gain an intellectual understanding about how you can develop unconditional self-acceptance, but you will not take many steps along the path to self-acceptance. You don't expect to learn how to play the piano just by reading a teach-yourself book on how to do it. You would expect that actually sitting down and playing the piano would form a central part of developing your expertise at this instrument. Well, exactly the same is true with learning self-acceptance. To learn it you have to practise it. This is a truism, of course, but it also happens to be true. So really be honest with yourself. You want to develop self-acceptance, but are you willing to spend some effort and energy in doing so? The decision, as the announcer on the TV programme *Blind Date* famously says, is yours.

Specify your self-depreciation problems

The very first step that you need to take along the path towards greater self-acceptance involves you specifying what problems you have in the realm of self-depreciation. Answering the following questions will help you do this. After I have listed each question I shall explain why answering it is important.

Question 1 *What do you put yourself down about?*

The first step in specifying your self-depreciation problems involves you identifying what kinds of events you put yourself down about (see pp. 3–7). When these events recur they are known as themes. Here are some examples of common themes that people typically depreciate themselves about:

- being criticized;
- being disliked/disapproved;
- not being loved;
- failing at important tasks;
- falling short (and often very short) of your ideals;
- being rejected;
- being fired from your job;
- breaking and/or failing to live up to your moral code;
- acting in socially inappropriate ways;
- regarding yourself as being overweight;
- regarding yourself as being unattractive;
- regarding yourself as having unappealing traits.

If you have what I call general unconditional self-depreciation you may well list all these themes, and more besides, because depreciating yourself is almost part of your identity. As one of my clients put it, 'I'm worthless because I am me. I dislike everything about myself.' If you suffer from general unconditional self-depreciation then I advise you to seek professional help, for you need more assistance than I can offer you in this book. Please see your doctor, who will suggest that you see a suitably qualified counsellor or psychotherapist. Having said this, you may still gain some benefit from reading this book and from carrying out the exercises that I will describe in the following chapters.

Question 2 *Taking each area listed below, how do you feel when you put yourself down?*

The second task in specifying your self-depreciation problems involves you identifying how you feel when you put yourself down (see pp. 1–3). Typically, when you depreciate yourself you will experience what are known as unhealthy negative emotions. The following is a list of such emotions:

- anxiety;
- depression;
- guilt;
- unhealthy anger;
- unhealthy jealousy;
- unhealthy envy;
- shame;
- hurt.

I suggest that you regard these emotions as signals that you may be depreciating yourself. I say 'may' here because you may experience some of these emotions for reasons other than self-depreciation.

Question 3 *When you put yourself down in each of the listed areas, what is the content of your self-depreciation?*

It is possible to depreciate yourself in many ways (see pp. 8–10). Here is an illustrative list:

- I am stupid;
- I am incompetent;
- I am insignificant;
- I am defective;
- I am pathetic;
- I am disgusting;
- I am worthless;
- I am a failure;
- I am a fool;
- I am no good;
- I am useless;
- I am weak;
- I am inferior;
- I am undeserving;
- I am bad/rotten;
- I am unlovable;

- I am unlikeable;
- I am second-rate;
- I am evil.

In addition, you may not think that you are worthless, for example, but you think that you are less worthy if you are criticized than if you are praised. Thus, some forms of self-depreciation reflect the fact that you think that you have some worth, but you can lose some of it if you are, in this instance, criticized.

Question 4 How do you act or 'feel' like acting once you have put yourself down for encountering situations described in your answer to Question 1?

Whenever you experience a significant emotion, you either act in certain ways or you feel an urge to act in those ways (known as action tendencies). It is important to gain an understanding of these actions and action tendencies because they often serve to maintain your self-depreciation problem, when the major emotion that you experience is negative and unhealthy (see above). Thus, if you feel hurt when you have been rejected, because you think that you are unlovable, you may hide away from others who can comfort you. If these others do not make an active attempt to seek you out (which they may not because they may think that your withdrawal means that you want to be on your own) then this may lead to your increased conviction that you are unlovable.

Question 5 Once you have put yourself down for encountering situations described in your answer to Question 1, how does this self-depreciation affect your subsequent thinking?

In the same way that self-depreciation influences the way you feel and act, it can also influence the way you subsequently think. Putting yourself down is equivalent to putting on a pair of bad sunglasses; it makes everything that you look at blacker and dimmer. Unless you understand this phenomenon you may regard your subsequent thinking as realistic rather than distorted by your negative opinion of yourself.

Question 6 How does your tendency to put yourself down in the areas you have specified in your answer to Question 1 affect the way you view situations when you encounter them, in reality or in imagination?

When you tend to depreciate yourself in certain areas (e.g. when you are criticized), this tendency leads you to be hypervigilant about the possibility of being criticized, even if your self-depreciation beliefs have not been fully activated. This often leads you to think in the following ways: it leads you to overestimate the likelihood that you will be criticized when this is a possibility; it leads you to infer that you have been criticized when in reality you have been given constructive feedback; and if you are criticized it leads you to exaggerate the extent of the criticism. Then, once you have constructed these inferences, you assume that they are true and these so-called events fully activate your self-depreciation beliefs.

Question 7 What steps do you take to avoid situations described in your answer to Question 1?

When you tend to depreciate yourself about a particular theme, e.g. failure, then you will tend to avoid these events. For example, you will not attempt a new task in case you fail at it and thus regard yourself as a failure. Avoiding threat is a basic human tendency which has two effects. First, it protects you from disturbing yourself in the very short term. Second, it strengthens your self-depreciation belief in the longer term. Thus, every time you avoid something in case you fail at it, you are rehearsing the idea that you are a failure should you fail.

Question 8 How do you compensate for your self-depreciation problems in each area listed in your answer to Question 1, and what effect does this compensation have?

When you compensate for a self-depreciation problem, you attempt to make good the damage you have done to your self (or are likely to do to your self). This often takes the form of doing something that diametrically opposes your depreciated view of yourself. A common example is a person who compensates for her view of herself as inferior by acting in a superior way. Another common compensatory strategy is found whenever you put someone else down in order to put yourself up the scale of worth that you have in your mind.

I will now show how Mandy, who I mentioned earlier in this chapter, answered the eight questions that I have just discussed. You might find it helpful to refer to Mandy's answers if you are unsure about the kinds of things to list in your answers.

An example of how to specify self-depreciation problems: the case of Mandy

Question 1:	What do you put yourself down about?
Answer (Mandy):	I put myself down when I am criticized and when other people seem to dislike me.

Question 2:   Taking each area listed above, how do you feel when you put yourself down?

Answer (Mandy):   When others criticize me, I feel hurt. I also feel anxious when I anticipate being criticized. When others dislike me, I feel depressed, and once again I also feel anxious when I anticipate others disliking me.

Question 3:   When you put yourself down in each of the listed areas, what is the content of your self-depreciation?

Answer (Mandy):   When I put myself down for being criticized, I think of myself as stupid, and when I put myself down for being disliked, I think of myself as worthless.

Question 4:   How do you act or 'feel' like acting once you have put yourself down for encountering situations described in your answer to Question 1?

Answer (Mandy):   When I am criticized and I think I am stupid, I make sure that I avoid the person who has criticized me. I also tend to sulk. When I think that someone does not like me and I consider myself to be worthless, I avoid that person if I can, or if not I go out of my way to be nice to them.

Question 5:   Once you have put yourself down for encountering situations described in your answer to Question 1, how does this self-depreciation affect your subsequent thinking?

Answer (Mandy):   When I think that I am stupid for being criticized I tend to think that I can do nothing right. When I think that I am worthless for being disliked, I think that no one will like me and that I will be alone.

Question 6:   How does your tendency to put yourself down in the areas you have specified in your answer to Question 1 affect the way you view situations when you encounter them in reality or in imagination?

Answer (Mandy): My tendency to think that I am stupid for being criticized leads me to think that I will be criticized unless I am perfect. My tendency to think that I am worthless for being disliked leads me to think that people will dislike me if I am not very nice to them.

Question 7: What steps do you take to avoid situations described in your answer to Question 1?

Answer (Mandy): To avoid being criticized I work very long hours so that nobody can find fault with what I do. I also go out of my way to be helpful to people who I see as particularly critical. Another thing that I do is to criticize myself first before anybody else has the chance to criticize me. This often has the effect of neutralizing any criticism the other person may have of me and they often reassure me that I am doing well. To avoid being disliked, I praise other people even though inwardly I don't think they have merited it. Also I show people that I like them and don't ever disagree with their opinions, even though privately I might hold very different opinions.

Question 8: How do you compensate for your self-deprecation problems in each area listed in your answer to Question 1, and what effect does this compensation have?

Answer (Mandy): To compensate for thinking that I am stupid when I am criticized, I criticize other people. I do this largely in my mind, but sometimes I do it out loud with people who I think are inferior to me. This has the effect of focusing my attention away from my own stupidity on to that of other people.

To compensate for thinking that I am worthless if people dislike me, I go out to make friends with new people. For everyone who doesn't like me, I feel that I have to make two new friends. This has the effect of getting rid of my feelings of worthlessness, at least temporarily.

In Table 1, I provide you with a list of the eight questions to ask yourself when specifying your self-depreciation problems. Why not take a photocopy of the list and carry it around with you so that when you have a spare moment you can reflect on the issues involved and write down relevant information? You will need to refer back to your answers as you proceed through the book.

Table 1   Specifying your self-depreciation problems

1 What do you put yourself down about?

2 Taking each area listed above, how do you feel when you put yourself down?

3 When you put yourself down in each of the listed areas, what is the content of your self-depreciation?

4 How do you act or 'feel' like acting once you have put yourself down for encountering situations described in your answer to Question 1?

5 Once you have put yourself down for encountering situations described in your answer to Question 1, how does this self-deprecia-tion affect your subsequent thinking?

6 How does your tendency to put yourself down in the areas you have specified in your answer to Question 1 affect the way you view situations when you encounter them?

7 What steps do you take to avoid situations described in your answer to Question 1?

8 How do you compensate for your self-depreciation problems in each are listed in your answer to Question 1, and what effect does this compensation have?

Setting goals

After you have specified your self-depreciation problems it is important that you be clear with yourself over what would be a realistic alternative to each of these problems. This is an important step, first because if you do not know where you are going you will not get there and second, because if you set an unrealistic goal then you will be easily discouraged when it becomes clear that you will not be able to achieve it.

As you do this goal-setting exercise it is important to be clear about the time-frame involved. When I run ten-week courses on developing self-acceptance I suggest that participants set goals that they think they can achieve by the end of the course. I stress that the course is designed to help participants acquire the knowledge and learn the skills to take the first steps towards unconditional self-acceptance and to know that regular practice of these skills is necessary to promote greater self-acceptance.

As a reader of this book, you can afford to be more ambitious in your goal setting since you are not limited to a ten-week course. Thus, I suggest that you take each self-depreciation problem that you specified in the previous section and set a realistic alternative as a goal for each problem. In doing this, you might find it helpful to use the same framework listed in Table 1 and illustrated in Mandy's response to the eight questions previously introduced and discussed. Let me first introduce you to and briefly discuss the goal framework, which I will then illustrate with reference to Mandy's goal statements.

Question 1 *What do you put yourself down about that you wish to accept yourself for?*

The answer to this question is obviously the same as it was when you specified your self-depreciation problems. The goal of self-acceptance training is to encourage you to accept yourself in the face of rejection, criticism, being disliked and all the themes that I listed on pp. 3–7, not to go out of your way to avoid them and to ensure that you live a life where such situations do not happen.

Question 2 *Taking each area listed above, what is healthy for you to feel instead of the unhealthy negative emotion listed in your specified problem?*

When you face a negative event about which you would normally put yourself down and experience an unhealthy negative emotion, it is unrealistic for you to work towards either feeling good about the event or feeling indifferent about it. Rather, it is realistic and constructive to work towards feeling healthily negative about the event. So when you accept yourself in the face of a negative event like being criticized or failing at an important task, expect to feel bad, but not disturbed. The following is a list of unhealthy negative emotions that you can experience when you depreciate yourself, and their healthy alternatives.

Unhealthy Negative Emotions (UNEs):	*Healthy Negative Emotions (HNEs):*
• anxiety	• concern
• depression	• sadness
• guilt	• remorse

39

- unhealthy anger
- unhealthy jealousy
- unhealthy envy
- shame
- hurt.

- healthy anger
- healthy jealousy
- healthy envy
- disappointment
- sorrow.

Question 3 In each area, how can you develop a self-accepting statement instead of a self-depreciating one?

You will recall from the previous chapter that the following are characteristics of unconditional self-acceptance. You are:

- human;
- alive;
- fallible;
- unique;
- too complex to be given a legitimate rating;
- in flux.

Thus, when you generate a self-acceptance statement, draw upon one or more of these characteristics. If you prefer to develop unconditional self-esteem where you regard yourself as worthy, unconditionally base your worth on the same characteristics since they will not change during your lifetime.

Question 4 What could you do once you have accepted yourself for encountering situations described in your answer to Question 1?

As I mentioned on p. 33, whenever you experience a significant emotion, you either act in certain ways or you feel an urge to act in those ways (known as action tendencies). When your major emotion is negative and healthy (see p. 23) and accompanies a self-accepting belief about a negative activating event, you will tend to act in ways that are constructive.

For example, I mentioned earlier that if you feel hurt (unhealthy negative emotion) when you have been rejected because you think that you are unlovable, you may hide away from others who can comfort you. However, if you accept yourself for being rejected and feel sorrow or regret (healthy negative emotion) about this, you will tend to seek comfort and solace from others and not sulk and withdraw. If you act constructively in response to situations where you would normally depreciate yourself, you will strengthen your conviction in your newly developed self-accepting belief and you will encourage a positive response from others which will also encourage you in this same regard.

Question 5 Once you have accepted yourself for encountering situations described in your answer to Question 1, how would this self-acceptance affect your subsequent thinking?

I mentioned earlier (see p. 33) that when you depreciate yourself your subsequent thinking tends to be distorted. In contrast, when you accept yourself your subsequent thinking tends to be realistic. For example, if you think you are stupid for failing at an important task and you think of attempting the task again, you will be more likely to overestimate the chances that you will fail again than you would if you had accepted yourself for your failure.

Question 6 How might accepting yourself unconditionally affect the way you view situations when you encounter them in reality or in imagination?

When you tend to depreciate yourself in a certain area you bring this tendency to situations that reflect this area, and this distorts the ways in which you view these situations (e.g. when you put yourself down for being criticized, this tendency leads you to be hypervigilant about the possibility of being criticized) even if your self-depreciation beliefs have not been fully activated. However, if you tend to accept yourself, this distorting effect is absent or much weaker than it is when you depreciate yourself and you tend to see these situations more objectively.

Thus, when you depreciate yourself in the face of criticism, you bring this tendency to situations where criticism is a possibility. For example, as mentioned earlier, you may: overestimate the likelihood that you will be criticized when this is a possibility; infer that you have been criticized when in reality you have been given constructive feedback; and, if you are criticized, your tendency to put yourself down leads you to exaggerate the extent of the criticism. However, when you accept yourself unconditionally for being criticized and you bring this tendency to situations where you may be criticized, then: you will be realistic in your view of the likelihood that you will be criticized when this is a possibility; if you have been given constructive feedback you will take it as such and not see it as criticism; and if you are criticized your tendency to accept yourself will lead you to see it for what it is, and you will thus not exaggerate its extent.

Question 7 What steps can you take to face situations described in your answer to Question 1?

You will not develop unconditional self-acceptance if you do not practise this philosophy while facing the situations you normally depreciate yourself about. Thus, if you tend to depreciate yourself for failing at important tasks, you may have developed sophisticated strategies for avoiding doing these tasks. Avoidance will not help to develop self-acceptance; rather, it is a significant impediment to your doing so. Thus, develop a sensible plan for facing up to those situations which you have depreciated yourself for in the past. As you do so, I suggest that you follow a principle I have called 'challenging, but not overwhelming'. This means that you face situations that you find challenging to confront but not (at that time) overwhelming.

Question 8 What can you constructively do instead of compensating for your self-depreciation problems in each area listed in your answer to Question 1?

If you recall, when you compensate for putting yourself down, you act in a way which involves you putting yourself up in your own mind. This may involve you doing something brilliantly well to compensate for the idea that you are stupid for doing something else poorly. Like avoidance, compensation serves to maintain your philosophy of self-depreciation because it is based on it. Instead of compensating for your self-depreciation problems, set yourself the goal of acting in ways that are based on the philosophy of unconditional self-acceptance.

Here is how Mandy answered these eight goal-oriented questions.

Question 1:	What do you put yourself down about that you wish to accept yourself for?
Answer (Mandy):	I put myself down when I am criticized and when other people seem to dislike me. My goal is to accept myself when this happens.
Question 2:	Taking each area listed above, what is healthy for you to feel instead of the unhealthy negative emotion listed in your specified problem?
Answer (Mandy):	When others criticize me, I feel hurt. Instead of feeling hurt it would be healthy for me to feel sorrowful when this happens. I also feel anxious when I anticipate being criticized and a healthier alternative to this would be to be concerned, but not anxious, about it.

When others dislike me, I currently feel depressed, and it would be healthier for me to feel sad instead. I also want to feel concerned instead of anxious when I anticipate others disliking me.

Question 3: In each area, how can you develop a self-accepting statement instead of a self-depreciating one?

Answer (Mandy): When I put myself down for being criticized, I think of myself as stupid. Instead, I could learn to think that I am a fallible person who acts well and stupidly, but I am not stupid through and through.

When I put myself down for being disliked, I think of myself as worthless. Instead, when I am disliked I can say that I am not worthless. My worth doesn't change whether I am liked or disliked.

Question 4: What could you do once you have accepted yourself for encountering situations described in your answer to question 1?

Answer (Mandy): I can face the person who has criticized me rather than avoid him or her. I can communicate to the person rather than sulk. When I think that someone does not like me I can check this out with them and discuss our respective feelings. Instead of going out of my way to be nice to them, I can act in a friendly way without being ingratiating, if I like the person. If I don't, I can be neutral to them.

Question 5: Once you have accepted yourself for encountering situations described in your answer to Question 1, how would this self-acceptance affect your subsequent thinking?

Answer (Mandy): Instead of thinking that I can do nothing right when I have or think that I have been criticized, I can learn to see that there are things I can do and things I can't. When someone dislikes me, instead of thinking that no one will like me and that I will be alone, I can take a balanced view

43

and see that some people will like me and others won't and that I will have periods of being on my own and periods of being with others.

Question 6:

How might accepting yourself unconditionally affect the way you view situations when you encounter them in reality or in imagination?

Answer (Mandy):

If I accept myself for any mistakes I make, then I am not linking criticism to not being perfect. Rather, I recognize that while some people will focus on what I haven't done right and criticize me for this, others will focus on what I have done right and compliment me on this.

If I accept myself for being disliked I am more likely to see that people will like and dislike me for many different reasons. People can still like me even if I do not go out of my way to be very nice to them.

Question 7:

What steps can you take to face situations described in your answer to Question 1?

Answer (Mandy):

On the issue of dealing with criticism, I can first make a list of people I find critical. Second, I can rank them in order from the least critical to the most critical, and then while practising my self-accepting beliefs I can show these people in rank order aspects of my work that are not that good, as long as doing so will not jeopardize my job.

I can also make a list of people who I think may not like me and rank them in order of how much I think they don't like me. Then I can work my way up the hierarchy and interact with them normally, without going out of my way to be nice to them, while practising accepting myself in the face of signs that they do not like me. In doing so, I will undertake to disagree with any of their opinions that I in fact disagree with.

Question 8:

What can you constructively do instead of compensating for your self-depreciation problems in each area listed in your answer to Question 1?

Answer (Mandy): Instead of criticizing others when I depreciate myself for doing something that I think I may be criticized for, I can work on accepting myself for my errors and accepting others for theirs. I will stop thinking others are inferior to me and, for that matter, superior to me.

If I do think that others dislike me, I will work on accepting myself for this and will not go out to make friends until I have done this.

In Table 2, I provide you with a list of the eight questions to ask yourself when setting goals with respect to your self-depreciation problems. Photocopy it and use it as a framework for your goal-setting. You will again need to refer back to your answers as you proceed through the book.

Table 2 Setting goals

---

1 What do you put yourself down about that you wish to accept yourself for?

2 Taking each area listed above, what is healthy for you to feel instead of the unhealthy negative emotion listed in your specified problem?

3 In each area, how can you develop a self-accepting statement instead of a self-depreciating one?

4 What could you do once you have accepted yourself for encountering situations described in your answer to Question 1?

5 Once you have accepted yourself for encountering situations described in your answer to Question 1, how would this self-acceptance affect your subsequent thinking?

6 How might accepting yourself unconditionally affect the way you view situations when you encounter them in reality or in imagination?

7 What steps can you take to face situations described in your answer to Question 1?

8 What can you constructively do instead of compensating for your self-depreciation problems in each area listed in your answer to Question 1?

In the next chapter, I will teach you how to analyse specific situations where you put yourself down. In particular I will focus on the unhealthy beliefs that underpin self-depreciation.

4

Analyse Your Self-depreciation Problems Using the ABC Framework

After you have specified your self-depreciation problems and have set realistic goals, the next step is for you to analyse or assess specific examples of these problems. In Rational Emotive Behaviour Therapy (the approach on which this book is based), and in other problem-oriented approaches to counselling, the first step to self-change is to begin with specific examples of more general problems. Once you have understood all the factors involved in specific self-depreciating episodes then you are better placed to help yourself in these specific episodes. Later, if you have been successful at self-help in the specific case you will be able to apply your learning more generally. So, in most cases I suggest that you work from the specific to the general in this book.

I recommend that you use REBT's ABC framework for analysing specific episodes of self-depreciation. Let me first deal with each element of the ABC framework in the order in which I suggest you use it in practice. However, there is one step to take before using the ABC framework, and this involves describing the situation in which you put yourself down.

Describe the situation in which you depreciated yourself

In using the ABC framework it is important to select a specific situation or episode to analyse. Once you have done so, you should describe the situation in which you depreciated yourself. Do so as specifically and as objectively as you can. However, don't worry at the moment if your description is distorted or biased. You will have an opportunity to learn how to spot and correct possible biases or distortions later in the book (see Chapter 6).

Mandy chose to analyse the following situation in which she depreciated herself. Here is her description of the event.

'I gave my boss the report and he focused on several spelling mistakes that I had made.'

Like Mandy, select a specific episode where you depreciated yourself, take a piece of paper and on the top write: 'Situation where I put myself down'. Describe this event as specifically and as objectively as you can under this heading.

C

In the ABC framework, C stands for the emotions, actions or action tendencies and thoughts that you had in response to your beliefs about the part of the event that you put yourself down for. This is why C stands for 'consequences' because they are consequences of your beliefs, which I will discuss presently.

Let me discuss the emotional, behavioural and thinking consequences of these beliefs in turn.

As I have already discussed, when you put yourself down it is very likely that you experience an unhealthy negative emotion. As I showed on pp. 1–3, this is likely to be anxiety, depression, guilt, shame, hurt, unhealthy anger, unhealthy jealousy and unhealthy envy. While you may experience more than one of these emotions in any particular self-depreciation episode, for the purpose of the analysis that you will be doing, select the main unhealthy negative emotion (or UNE), if indeed you experience more than one, and write this down under the heading 'C (emotional)' on your piece of paper (see Table 3 on pp. 50–51).

As you can see from Mandy's form (reproduced in Table 3) her major UNE was depression.

When you put yourself down it is likely that you act in a certain way or experience an urge to act in a certain way (this latter urge is known as an action tendency). Most often, when you depreciate yourself your actions or action tendencies are likely to be unconstructive and self-defeating. You list these next to 'C (behavioural)' on your sheet.

As you can see from Table 3, Mandy listed 'withdrawal into myself' as her actual behavioural consequence.

The final set of consequences that I want to discuss is known as thinking consequences. This refers to how you think once you are in a self-depreciating frame of mind. This is different from the type of thinking (known as beliefs) you engage in that led you to put yourself down in the first place. I will discuss these beliefs when I consider the B section of the ABC framework below. The thinking consequences of holding beliefs at B are placed under the heading 'C (thinking)' in the ABC framework. When you depreciate yourself, your subsequent thinking is likely to be negative, exaggerated and distorted.

As can be seen from Table 3, Mandy said that her self-depreciation about what her boss said led her subsequently to think that she would never be able to please him and led her to focus on what she did wrong rather than what she did right.

You may be wondering at this point why I suggest that you begin with C when you use the ABC framework. The reason for this is that C factors, and in particular your emotions, are frequently the first things you are aware of when you put yourself down. They also serve as good signposts to what you feel most disturbed about at A in the ABC framework (which I will discuss in the next section). However, the REBT model is a flexible approach to self-help and, as such, you may at times find it more useful to begin your analysis of your chosen specific episode by identifying A, to which I now turn.

A

In the REBT model A stands for an activating event. In the episode that you have chosen to analyse, there are potentially several different activating events that you can focus on. You can focus on the content of what someone says to you, for example, the tone in which they say it, their body language or several other factors in the situation. However, your task at this point is to identify the aspect of the situation about which you depreciated yourself. This is known as the critical A and, looking at it slightly differently, it is the feature of the situation that you felt most disturbed about.

One way of identifying the critical A is to attempt to do so at one go. Here you can ask yourself one (or both) of the following questions:

1 What was the aspect of the situation that I put myself down most about?
2 What was the aspect of the situation that I was most disturbed about?

If asking these questions does not help you to find the critical A, you might find it helpful to use another technique, known as inference chaining. I will now outline the steps that you need to take when using inference chaining and will illustrate the method by showing how Mandy employed it.

1 Begin by taking the unhealthy negative emotion (UNE) you identified at point C in the ABC framework (see above).

Mandy's UNE, if you recall, was depression.

2 Ask yourself the question: 'What did I find depressing (or anxiety-provoking, or whatever was your major UNE) about the situation that I found myself in (as described earlier)?'

Mandy asked herself: 'What was depressing about my boss focusing on the spelling mistakes that I made in the report that I gave him?' Her reply was: 'He thinks I am incompetent.'

3 When you respond to the above question, assume temporarily that your response is true. You will have an opportunity of questioning how true it is later. Treating your response as if it were true at this point helps you to identify the critical A in the episode under consideration.

So, taking this response, ask yourself the question: 'And what did I find most depressing (or whatever emotion was experienced) about that?'

Mandy asked herself: 'What did I find was most depressing about my boss thinking that I was incompetent?' Her response was: 'If my boss thinks that I am incompetent this proves I am not capable of impressing him.'

4 Continue in this vein until you have identified your critical A. How do you know that you have identified your critical A? The following are signs that your A is critical:

- You know once you have identified an A that this was the aspect of the situation that you most depreciated yourself for.
- You mention a self-depreciating belief in your response.
- You begin to experience the same emotion that you listed under C when you have identified the A.
- You cannot think of any other aspect of the situation that you put yourself down for when you ask yourself the question: 'And what did I find most depressing (or whatever emotion was experienced) about that?'

Mandy continued as follows:

Question: 'And what was most depressing about not being able to impress my boss?'

Answer: 'If I can't impress my boss this proves that I am incompetent as a person.' At this point Mandy began to feel depressed and as you can see she articulated a self-depreciating belief: 'I am incompetent as a person.' These two signs meant that she had probably identified her critical A which was: 'Not being able to impress my boss'.

Once you have identified your critical A, write it down on your piece of paper under the heading 'A'.

B

When you depreciate or put yourself down, you generally hold two types of belief. First, you hold a rigid demand about yourself, other people and/or the world. Then, you tend to give yourself a global negative rating of your self. According to the ABC framework, your demanding beliefs and your negative ratings of your self when you hold such beliefs about critical activating events are at the core of your self-depreciation problems.

Mandy's beliefs about not being able to impress her boss (i.e. her critical A) were as follows: 'I must be able to impress my boss' and 'I'm worthless if I am not able to impress my boss.' These beliefs led Mandy to feel depressed in this episode.

Table 3 Mandy's ABC

Situation in which I put myself down: 'I gave my boss the report and he focused on several spelling mistakes that I had made.'

A (critical) =	'I'm not capable of impressing my boss'
B (demand) =	'I must be able to impress my boss'
(self depreciating belief) =	'I'm a failure if I can't impress my boss'

C (emotional) =   Depressed

  (behavioural) =   Withdrawal into myself

  (thinking) =   'I will never be able to please my boss'

                                    'I focused on what I did wrong rather than on what I did right'

General instructions for completing the ABC form

Table 4 details a blank form which you may find useful as a framework when you analyse specific examples of your self-depreciation. Here is a set of step-by-step instructions for you to follow when completing this form.

Step 1   Select a specific example where you depreciated yourself and describe this situation as clearly and as objectively as you can.

Step 2   Identify your major emotion, your major action or action tendency and how you subsequently thought, and write these down next to the headings C (emotional), C (behavioural) and C (thinking) respectively.

Step 3   Identify what you were most disturbed about in the episode under consideration (or what you most put yourself down for). Use your identified emotional C to do an inference chain if you need to. Write down your critical A next to A (critical) on the form.

Step 4   Identify the demand and the self-depreciation belief that you held about A which resulted in your response at C. Put the demand next to B (demand) and the self-depreciation belief next to B (self-depreciation belief).

Table 4 ABC form

Situations in which I put myself down:

A (critical) =

B (demand) =

   (self-depreciation belief) =

C (emotional) =

   (behavioural) =

   (thinking) =

I suggest that you use the ABC form on several occasions so that you develop competence at analysing specific episodes where you depreciated yourself. Once you have done this, you are ready to go on to the next step in developing self-acceptance, which is questioning the unhealthy beliefs that underpin your self-depreciation and the beliefs that underpin self-acceptance. This is the focus of the next chapter.

5

Question Your Beliefs

The Rational Emotive Behaviour Therapy model upon which this book is based argues that two unhealthy beliefs are at the core of your self-depreciation problems: demands and self-depreciation beliefs. I discussed these two unhealthy beliefs in Chapter 2. REBT also states that two beliefs are at the core of the healthy alternative to self-depreciation, known as the philosophy of unconditional self-acceptance. These two beliefs are full preferences and self-acceptance beliefs. I also discussed these two beliefs in Chapter 2.

When you come to analyse specific examples where you put yourself down, one of your major tasks is to identify the demands and self-depreciating beliefs which mediate between the event and your disturbed responses to the event. I showed you how to do this in the previous chapter. Once you have done this it is important that you identify the healthy alternatives to these beliefs. I will cover this topic in the present chapter. After doing this you then have a choice: to maintain your conviction in your unhealthy beliefs or to work towards gaining conviction in your healthy beliefs. Before you decide which of these two courses of action you wish to take, it is important that you question both sets of beliefs so that you can make an informed choice to commit yourself to one or the other. Questioning your beliefs is the major focus of the present chapter. But first, let me discuss healthy alternatives to the unhealthy beliefs that underpin your self-depreciation problems.

Identify the healthy alternatives to demands and self-depreciation beliefs

The healthy alternative to a demand that underpins a self-depreciation problem is known as a full preference. When you hold a full preference you assert what you want, but acknowledge that your desire does not have to be fulfilled. Let me illustrate this with reference to Mandy's demand listed in Table 3 (see pp. 51–52). As you can see from this table, Mandy's demand in the episode that she chose to analyse was: 'I must be able to impress my boss.' Mandy's full preference alternative to this demand is: 'I want to be able to impress my boss, but I do not have to do so.' This belief is a full preference because it asserts what Mandy wants (i.e. 'I want to be able to impress my boss . . .') and it negates her demand (i.e. '. . . but I do not have to do so'). The distinction between a demand and a full preference is important and I suggest that you make a note of it before reading the next section of this chapter.

The healthy alternative to a self-depreciating belief is known as a self-accepting belief. When you hold a self-accepting belief, you *both* assert that you are a fallible human being who is too complex to merit a single rating (or similar variant) *and* negate the global self-rating that you gave yourself in your self-depreciating belief. Let me again illustrate this with reference to Mandy's example. In Table 3 Mandy's self-depreciating belief is listed as: 'I am a failure if I can't impress my boss.' Mandy's self-acceptance belief alternative to this belief is: 'I am not a failure. I am a fallible human being who is not able to impress by boss.' This belief is a self-acceptance belief because it asserts who Mandy is (a fallible human being who is not able to please) and it negates who Mandy is not – she is not a failure.

How to question your beliefs

After you have specified the healthy alternatives to your demands and self-depreciation beliefs, you are now ready to question your beliefs. When you do so I suggest that you question your demands and full preferences together and your self-depreciation beliefs and self-acceptance beliefs together. I also suggest that you ask yourself four questions of each set of beliefs:

- Which belief is true and which is false?
- Which belief is logical and which is illogical?
- Which belief is helpful and which is unhelpful?
- Which belief do you wish to strengthen and act on?

Let me now illustrate how Mandy questioned one of her demands and full preferences and one of her self-depreciation beliefs and self-acceptance beliefs.

How Mandy questioned her demand and full preference

I will start with how Mandy questioned her demand and full preference about impressing her boss.

First, Mandy wrote down her demand and full preference next to each other on a sheet of paper under the appropriate headings:

Demand	*Full preference*
'I must be able to impress my boss.'	'I want to be able to impress my boss, but I do not have to do so.'

Second, Mandy asked herself the question: 'Which of these two beliefs is true and which is false?'

Third, Mandy's answer was as follows: My demand is false and my full preference is true. My demand is false because if there was a law of the universe which decreed that I must be able to impress my boss, I would not have to worry about this issue since I would have to impress my boss. He would be a puppet because he would be obligated to be impressed by me. Obviously no such demand exists.

On the other hand, my full preference is true. It is true that I want to be able to impress my boss and it is also true that I do not have to do so.

Fourth, Mandy asked herself the question: 'Which belief is sensible/logical and which doesn't make sense or is illogical?

Fifth, Mandy answered this question as follows? My demand is illogical because while I may want to be able to impress my boss, it is illogical for me to conclude that therefore I have to be able to do so. The first part of this statement: 'I want to impress my boss' is flexible, while the second part of this statement: 'and therefore I have to be able to do so' is rigid, and you can't logically derive a rigidity from something that is flexible.

On the other hand, my full preference is sensible. It makes sense to say that while I may want to be able to impress my boss, I do not have to do so. Both parts of this statement are flexible and are thus logically connected together.

Sixth, Mandy asked herself the question: 'Which belief is helpful and yields healthy results, and which is unhelpful and yields unhealthy results?'

Seventh, Mandy answered this question as follows: My demand is unhelpful because I will be anxious in case I am not able to impress my boss and depressed when it becomes clear to me that I can't impress him. This demand will also lead me to act and think in unhealthy ways. Thus, I may go out of my way to impress him instead of concentrating on the job at hand. I also may give up trying to do a good job once it becomes apparent that I can't impress my boss.

On the other hand, my full preference is helpful because I will feel concerned, but not anxious, in case I am not able to impress my boss, and will feel sad or disappointed, but not depressed, when it is clear that I cannot do so. This full preference will also lead me to act and think in constructive ways. Thus, I will be able to concentrate on what I am doing rather than on how well I am doing, and I will consequently be more effective in my work. I will also continue to do a good job even though I am unable to impress my boss because I will be doing a good job for myself and not just for him.

Eighth, Mandy asked herself the following question: 'Which of the two beliefs do I want to strengthen and act on?'

Ninth, Mandy answered this question as follows: I want to strengthen and act on my full preference because it will lead me to be more inner directed in my work and stop me from obsessing about how my boss is reacting to my work. It will also lead me to enjoy my work more because at the moment, with my need to impress my boss, I am living in a constant state of anxiety at work which is definitely interfering with my ability to enjoy what I do at work.

How Mandy questioned her self-depreciation and self-acceptance beliefs

Now let me present how Mandy questioned her self-depreciating and self-accepting beliefs about failing to impress her boss.

First, Mandy wrote down her self-depreciation belief and her self-acceptance belief next to each other on a sheet of paper under the appropriate headings:

Self-depreciation belief	*Self-acceptance belief*
'I am a failure if I can't impress my boss.'	'If I am not able to impress my boss I am not a failure. I am a fallible human being who has failed in this respect.'

Second, Mandy asked herself the question: 'Which of these beliefs is true and which is false?'

Third, Mandy's answer was as follows: My self-depreciation belief is false and my self-acceptance belief is true. My self-depreciation is false because I can prove that I am not a failure. If I were a failure then I could not succeed at anything, either now, in the past or in the future. This is patently nonsense.

On the other hand, my self-acceptance belief is true because I can prove that I am fallible for failing to be able to impress my boss. Being fallible means being able to succeed at some things and to fail at others. This is a very accurate description of myself.

Fourth, Mandy asked herself the question: 'Which belief is sensible/logical and which doesn't make sense or is illogical?'

Fifth, Mandy answered this question as follows: My self-depreciation belief is illogical because it makes no logical sense for me to say that because I am not able to impress my boss this proves that I am a failure. In making this statement I am committing the part–whole error which falsely assumes that you can rate the whole on the basis of one or more of its parts, when logically you can do no such thing.

On the other hand, my self-acceptance belief does make sense because it is logical for me to say that because I am unable to impress my boss this proves that I am a fallible human being who can succeed at some things and fail at others. Here I am saying that as a fallible human being I can succeed and fail. This logically follows on from the statement that I have failed in the aspect of impressing my boss.

Sixth, Mandy asked herself the question: 'Which belief is helpful and yields healthy results and which is unhelpful and yields unhealthy results?'

Seventh, Mandy answered this question as follows: My self-depreciation belief is unhelpful because once again it will lead me to be anxious in case I am not able to impress him and depressed once it becomes clear to me that I cannot do so. Putting myself down in this way will also lead me to act and think in unhealthy ways. Since I am basing my worth on my ability to impress my boss, I will place too much emphasis on this and will do what I think he wants me to do instead of doing what I think it is right to do. This will interfere with my ability to think creatively and independently at work, which I am paid to do, and will lead me to play safe.

On the other hand, my self-acceptance belief is helpful because I will again feel concerned, but not anxious, in case I am not able to impress my boss and will feel sad or disappointed, but not depressed, once it becomes apparent that I cannot impress him. This self-acceptance belief will also lead me to act and think in constructive ways. I will be able to concentrate on the task at hand and do what I think is right instead of constantly asking myself whether my boss will be impressed.

Eighth, Mandy asked herself the following question: 'Which of the two beliefs do I want to strengthen and act on?'

Ninth, Mandy answered this question as follows: I want to strengthen and act on my self-acceptance belief because it will benefit me in so many ways. It will help me to enjoy my job and lead me to take healthy, considered risks rather than playing safe. It will help me to tell my boss when I think he is making the wrong decision and it will enable me to suggest ways in which I think we can improve things in the office which my boss may not agree with.

Questioning your demands and full preferences

In Table 5 I present a form which I suggest you use when you come to question your demands and full preferences.

Table 5 Questioning demands and full preferences

Step 1 Take your demand and identify the alternative full preference to this belief. Write them side by side on a sheet of paper under the following headings.

| *Demand* | *Full preference* |

Step 2 Ask yourself the question 'Which belief is true and which is false?'

Step 3 Write down the answer to this question and provide written reasons for your answer.

Step 4 Ask yourself the question 'Which belief is sensible/logical and which doesn't make sense or is illogical?'

Step 5 Write down the answer to this question and provide written reasons for your answer.

Step 6 Ask yourself the question 'Which belief is helpful/yields healthy results and which is unhelpful/yields unhealthy results?'

Step 7 Write down the answer to this question and provide written reasons for your answer.

Step 8 Ask yourself the question 'Which of the two beliefs do you want to strengthen and act on?'

Step 9 Write down the answer to this question and provide written reasons for your answer.

Let me now alert you to some typical difficulties that people have with the different steps on this form and how you can avoid them.

Step 1 Specify your demand and full preference

The main difficulty that you are likely to experience at this initial step is failing to specify your full preference. Thus, instead of stating that your full preference is, for example, 'I want to do well at my forthcoming interview, but I don't have to do so', you might write: 'I want to do well at my forthcoming interview', which is a partial preference. A partial preference is a statement of a preference without the demand being negated. The problem with stating a partial preference is that it does not negate your demand. Consequently, if you remain with your partial preference, you may later transform this into a demand: 'Because I want to do well at my forthcoming interview, therefore I have to do so.' However, if you specify your full preference, you are far less likely to transform this into a demand because in a full preference you are explicitly negating your demand: 'I want to do well at my forthcoming interview, BUT I don't have to do so.' So, in specifying your full preference, assert your preference: 'I want to do well at my forthcoming interview . . .' AND negate your demand: '. . . BUT I do not have to do so'.

Step 3 Write down the answer to the question: 'Which belief is true and which is false?' and provide written reasons for your answer

If you find answering this question difficult it is useful to bear in mind the following:

1 Your full preference is true for the following reasons: First, it is true because you can prove that you have it. Your desire is your desire. Second, it is true because you can prove why you have your preference. And third, it is true because you can prove that you don't have to have your desire met.

   Thus, your full preference that you want to do well in your forthcoming interview, but that you don't have to do so is true for the following reasons: First, it is true because you can prove that you have a desire to do well in your forthcoming interview. Second, it is true because you can prove why you want to do well in this circumstance. And third, it is true because you can prove that you don't have to do well in the interview.

2 Your demand is false, because if it were true then whatever you were demanding would have to exist. It could not fail to exist. As there

exists the possibility that whatever you are demanding may not exist, your demand is not consistent with reality.

Thus, your demand that you must do well in your forthcoming interview is false, because if it were true then you would have to do well in the interview. You could not fail to do well in this circumstance. As there exists the possibility that you may not do well in the interview, your demand is not consistent with reality.

Step 5 Write down the answer to the question: 'Which belief is sensible/logical and which doesn't make sense or is illogical?' and provide written reasons for your answer

If you find answering this question difficult, the following may help:

1 Take your partial preference.
  (Using our example: 'I want to do well in my forthcoming interview.')
2 Recognize that you can transform this partial preference into either a full preference or a demand.
  ('I want to do well in my forthcoming interview, but I do not have to do so.')
  'I want to do well in my forthcoming interview, and therefore I have to do so.')
3 Realize that your full preference logically follows from your partial preference because both are flexible.
  ('I want to do well in my forthcoming interview [partial preference – flexible] but I do not have to do so [full preference – flexible].')
4 Realize that your demand does not follow logically from your partial preference, because the former is inflexible and the latter is flexible and something inflexible cannot sensibly follow on from something flexible.
  ('I want to do well in my forthcoming interview [partial preference – flexible] and therefore I have to do so [demand – inflexible].')

Step 7 Write down the answer to the question: 'Which belief is helpful/yields healthy results and which is unhelpful/yields unhealthy results?' and provide written reasons for your answer

A common misconception here is that you may think that your demand motivates you and that your full preference leads to resignation. While there may be a grain of truth to this argument it is largely untrue. Thus, while demands can be motivating, they are frequently motivating in unproductive ways. In particular, demands impair objective decision-making and thus your actions are unduly influenced by the disturbed emotions that often stem from rigid demands (see p. 14). For example, anxiety-related demands can be motivating, but you tend to behave in a frantic, directionless way, like a headless chicken.

In contrast, full preferences are motivating because they indicate what you want. However, this motivation is far more likely to be based on careful thought since you acknowledge that you don't have to have your desire met. So the first part of a full preference (e.g. 'I want to do well in my forthcoming interview . . .') propels you forward towards doing well at the interview, and the second part (e.g. '. . . but I don't have to do so') ensures that this forward propulsion is not influenced by emotional disturbance.

Demands are, in fact, more likely than full preferences to lead to resignation. This is because you are more likely to conclude that you will never achieve your goal when your demand is not met than when your full preference is not met. Holding this latter belief is likely to lead to a realistic appraisal of your chances of achieving your goal, and this realistic appraisal is likely to encourage persistent striving towards that goal. This is the antithesis of resignation.

In summary, while full preferences may not foster the frantic, mindless type of motivation that some might find appealing because of the immediate buzz that this gives, they often promote a steadier, considered type of motivation which, in the longer term, is likely to produce better results for you than the frantic, mindless motivation stimulated by demands.

Questioning your self-depreciation and self-acceptance beliefs

In Table 6, I present a form which I suggest you use when you come to question your self-depreciation and self-acceptance beliefs.

Table 6 Questioning self-depreciation beliefs and self-acceptance beliefs

---

Step 1 Take your self-depreciation belief and identify the alternative self-acceptance belief. Write them side by side on a sheet of paper under the following headings.

Self-depreciation belief	*Self-acceptance belief*

Step 2 Ask yourself the question 'Which belief is true and which is false?'

Step 3 Write down the answer to this question and provide written reasons for your answer.

Step 4 Ask yourself the question 'Which belief is sensible/logical and which doesn't make sense or is illogical?'

Step 5 Write down the answer to this question and provide written reasons for your answer.

Step 6 Ask yourself the question 'Which belief is helpful/yields healthy results and which is unhelpful/yields unhealthy results?'

Step 7 Write down the answer to this question and provide written reasons for your answer.

Step 8 Ask yourself the question 'Which of the two beliefs do you want to strengthen and act on?'

Step 9 Write down the answer to this question and provide written reasons for your answer.

Let me again alert you to some typical difficulties that people have with the different steps on this form and how you can avoid them.

Step 1 Specify your self-depreciation belief and your self-acceptance belief

You may experience two difficulties with this step. First, you may fail to specify a true self-depreciation belief. Instead you may put forward a statement in which you rate one of your traits (e.g. 'I am selfish') or one of your roles (e.g. 'I am a bad mother').

If you have put forward a trait masquerading as a self-rating, you are using an adjective which is a trait and not a rating of your entire self. Thus, if you say 'I am selfish' the term 'selfish' refers to a trait (i.e. selfishness). The self-rating here is something like 'I am less worthy for being selfish.'

The same is true when you put forward a role masquerading as a self-rating (e.g. 'I am a bad mother'). Thus, 'mother' is clearly a role that you occupy and is not equivalent to your entire self. The self-rating here is something like 'I am a bad person if I am a bad mother.'

Thus, whenever your self-rating is really a trait rating or a role rating, look for the implicit self-rating and write it on the form under the heading 'self-depreciation belief'.

The second difficulty that you may experience with this step is failing to provide a full self-acceptance belief. For example, let's suppose you say: 'I am not a failure if I do not do well in my forthcoming interview.' This statement is what may be called a partial self-acceptance belief in that you state who you are not (in this case a failure). By contrast, a full self-acceptance belief states who you are not: 'I am not a failure if I do not do well in my forthcoming interview' and asserts who you are: 'I am a fallible human being who has not done well on this occasion. My worth as a person doesn't change, no matter what I do.'

Thus, provide a full self-acceptance belief, otherwise you may transform a partial self-acceptance belief ('I am not a failure if I don't do well in my forthcoming interview') into a subtle self-depreciation belief ('. . . but I would be worthier if I did well than if I didn't').

Step 3 Write down the answer to the question: 'Which belief is true and which is false?' and provide written reasons for your answer

If you find answering this question difficult it is useful to bear in mind the following:

1 Your self cannot be rated on the basis of what you do or on the basis of one or more of your characteristics. It is far too complex for that.

  Thus, if it were true that you were a failure for doing poorly at your forthcoming interview, then you would fail at everything that you do, since 'I am a failure' means that this is your essence. This is false, since a moment's reflection will indicate to you that you have succeeded at things as well as failed.

2 On the other hand, you can prove that you are a fallible human being because this is your essence as a person.

  Thus, is it true that you are a fallible human being for failing to do well at your forthcoming interview, for being fallible means having the capacity to do poorly at things as well as doing well at them.

Step 5 Write down the answer to the question: 'Which belief is sensible/logical and which doesn't make sense or is illogical?' and provide written reasons for your answer

If you find answering this question difficult, the following may help:

1 Take the event at A (pp. 49–51), or the aspect of the A about which you were most disturbed (i.e. your critical A).

  (Not doing well at your forthcoming interview)

2 Realize that when you rate your self negatively on the basis of this event, or critical A, you are making an illogical part–whole error where you think that you can rate the whole of your self on the basis of one of your experiences or on the basis of your behaviour or one of your characteristics.

(I am a failure [whole defined by part] for not doing well at the interview [part]. This belief is based on the part–whole error and thus is illogical.)

3 Realize that when you do not rate your self but accept yourself as a fallible human being for what has occurred at A, then this makes sense because your self can incorporate A without being defined by it.

('If I do not do well at my forthcoming interview [part], I am not a failure. I am a fallible human being who has not done well on this occasion [incorporates part without being defined by it]. This is sensible because I am not making the part–whole error.)

Step 7 Write down the answer to the question: 'Which belief is helpful/yields healthy results and which is unhelpful/yields unhealthy results?' and provide written reasons for your answer

In general, you can probably see that self-depreciation beliefs lead to unhealthy results and self-acceptance beliefs lead to healthy results. However, as with demands and full preferences, you may think that self-depreciation beliefs have motivational properties and that self-acceptance beliefs promote resignation. The points that I made when addressing this misconception with respect to demands and full preferences are relevant here as well. For example, if you think that your self-depreciation belief (e.g. 'I am a failure') stimulates productive change, consider this: if you think that you are a failure, then what does a failure do other than fail? As such, when you are faced with performing an important task and you think you are a failure, you will be less rather than more likely to persist at that task. On the other hand, if you accept yourself as a fallible human being who can succeed as well as fail, you are more likely to persist at the important task than when you consider yourself to be a failure. This is because this self-acceptance belief will lead you to think that you have as much chance of succeeding at the task as of failing at it.

The purpose of questioning your beliefs

The main initial purpose of questioning your beliefs in the way I have suggested is the acquisition of intellectual insight. This means that at the end of this questioning process, which has to be done repeatedly and not just once in a while, you will understand intellectually that your demands and self-depreciation beliefs are false, illogical and largely unhelpful, and that your full preferences and self-acceptance beliefs are true, sensible and largely helpful. You will not yet have developed strong conviction in your full preferences and self-acceptance beliefs so that they will help you to feel healthy emotions, to act constructively or to think realistically, but you will have laid down important foundations that will help you to develop strong conviction in your healthy beliefs later. In order to develop emotional insight – which in this context means that you will understand deeply that your demands and self-depreciation beliefs are false, illogical and largely unhelpful and that your full preferences and self-acceptance beliefs are true, sensible and largely helpful and that this understanding will have a profound influence on the way you feel, act and subsequently think – you will have to perform a variety of other tasks, again repeatedly, which I will outline in the remainder of this book.

6

Strengthen Your Conviction in Your Healthy Beliefs

In the previous chapter, I showed you how to question your beliefs, the purpose of which was for you to understand intellectually why your demands and self-depreciation beliefs are inconsistent with reality, illogical and largely unhelpful and why your full preferences and self-acceptance beliefs are consistent with reality, sensible and largely helpful. However, to really change your beliefs you need to do more than question them in the way that I described. In this chapter, I will teach you four techniques which will help you to strengthen your conviction in your healthy beliefs (i.e. your full preferences and self-acceptance beliefs). But first, let me explain the process of belief change.

The process of belief change

If you understand how belief change happens then you will be prepared to put into practice the principles and techniques that I will cover in the remainder of this book. So here is an account of the process of belief change.

1 Belief change involves weakening unhealthy beliefs and strengthening healthy beliefs. You have laid the foundations for this by learning to question your demands and self-depreciation beliefs on the one hand and your full preferences and self-acceptance beliefs on the other. You will continue this process by using the techniques that I will teach you in this chapter.

2 As you strengthen your healthy beliefs and weaken your unhealthy beliefs, it is very likely that you will experience a strong sense of discomfort. This discomfort is due to the fact that you are used to your unhealthy beliefs and are unused to your healthy beliefs. In order to consolidate your belief change you need to tolerate this discomfort while continuing this weakening–strengthening process.

3 As you do so, it is very important that you begin to act in accord with your healthy beliefs (i.e. your full preferences and self-acceptance beliefs) and refrain from acting in accord with your unhealthy beliefs (i.e. your demands and self-depreciation beliefs). If you change your thinking in the direction of your healthy beliefs but keep acting in

accord with your unhealthy beliefs, you will undermine the belief change process.

4 You will facilitate the belief change process if you frequently practise thinking and acting in accord with your healthy beliefs.

5 You will facilitate the belief change process if you add force, energy and passion to this process. This means strongly rehearsing your healthy beliefs rather than doing so in a weak, wimpish manner. It also means acting in accord with your healthy beliefs in a whole-hearted manner rather than doing so tentatively.

6 If you stop acting and thinking in accord with your healthy beliefs, you will increase the chances of returning to your unhealthy beliefs. Thus, you would be wise to make a long-term commitment to act and think in accord with your developing self-acceptance philosophy.

The following thinking-based techniques have been devised to help you to strengthen your conviction in your full preferences and self-acceptance beliefs. In the following chapter, I will describe a number of action-based techniques which have the same purpose.

The rational portfolio technique

A rational portfolio contains a range of arguments in favour of a healthy belief and against an unhealthy belief. In developing a rational portfolio for yourself, think of as many arguments as you can why your full preferences and self-acceptance beliefs are true, sensible and constructive and why your demands and self-depreciation beliefs are false, illogical and unconstructive. The idea is to swamp yourself with arguments in favour of your healthy belief and against your unhealthy belief. You may think that this shows bias, but don't forget that you have already determined why your demands and self-depreciation beliefs are unhealthy and why your full preferences and self-acceptance beliefs are healthy. The rational portfolio takes this idea and builds upon it.

Table 7 outlines the rational portfolio constructed by Fiona, a member of one of my 'Developing Self-acceptance' groups.

Table 7 Fiona's rational portfolio

Unhealthy belief	*Healthy belief*
'The woman at the party must like me. If she doesn't then I'm worthless.'	'I'd like the woman at the party to like me, but she doesn't have to do so. If she doesn't like me then I am not worthless. Rather, I am a fallible human being who is not liked by the woman in question.'
Reasons why this belief is unhealthy:	Reasons why this belief is healthy:
1 There is no law of the universe which states that the woman at the party must like me. If there was such a law, she would have to like me.	1 My full preference is true because I am indicating the truth of my desire, i.e. I want the woman at the party to like me.
2 When I demand that the woman at the party must like me, I deprive her of her free will. As she is a person, she has the freedom to dislike me if that's how she feels.	2 My full preference is also true because I am recognizing that there is no law of the universe which states that the woman at the party must like me.
3 Demanding that the woman at the party must like me is illogical because this demand does not logically follow from what I want – which is for her to like me. A demand does not logically follow from a preference.	3 By wanting the woman at the party to like me, but not demanding that she must do so, I am recognizing that she has free will. I am acknowledging that as a person she has the freedom to dislike me if that's how she feels.
4 If the woman does not like me, this is a fact and therefore it is just not sensible for me to demand that she likes me.	4 My acknowledgement that the woman at the party does not have to like me follows logically from my desire that I would like her to do so.

5 If the woman at the party dislikes me, then again this is a fact and when I demand that she must like me, I am insisting that reality must not be reality, which is crazy.

5 If the woman at the party does not like me, this is a fact, and therefore it is sensible for me to indicate that she does not have to like me.

6 Demanding that the woman at the party must like me will lead me to be anxious before I conclude that she doesn't like me, and depressed when I draw that conclusion.

6 If the woman at the party dislikes me, then again this is a fact, and when I state that I want her to like me, but she doesn't have to do so, I am acknowledging that reality does not have to be different from the way that it is, although I would like it to be so.

7 When I demand that the woman must like me, this demand will result in my trying desperately to get her to like me. When I act desperately, I probably increase the chances that she won't like me or if she does she won't be liking *me*, but the false image that I portray.

7 Preferring, but not demanding, that the woman at the party like me will lead me to be concerned, but not anxious, before I conclude that she doesn't like me, and sad, but not depressed, after I have drawn this conclusion. Concern and sadness are healthy negative emotions because they help me to face up to a negative life event without disturbing myself about it.

8 Even if the woman at the party likes me for myself, demanding that she must like me will render me anxious in case she dislikes me later.

8 When I prefer the woman to like me, but do not demand that she must do so, this full preference will not result in my trying desperately to get her to like me. I might try to get her to like me, but I will not do so in a desperate manner. My lack of desperation

will increase the chances that she will like me and that she will like me for myself and not for any false act that I may put on.

9 When I demand that the woman at the party must like me, I will tend to assume that she doesn't like me unless she shows clear evidence that she likes me. Thus, if she likes me a little or is neutral towards me then the absence of clear evidence that she likes me will lead me to conclude wrongly that she dislikes me.

9 If the woman at the party likes me, my full preference will lead me to be concerned, but not anxious, about the prospect that she may dislike me later.

10 When I conclude that I am worthless if the woman at the party dislikes me, then I am making a false statement. For as a person I cannot be rated. Rather, I am a fallible human being who is unrateable. Even if I have worth, this worth cannot be taken away by her dislike of me. I am worthwhile because I am human, unique and alive and not because the woman at the party likes me.

10 When I want the woman at the party to like me, but do not demand that she has to do so, I will not automatically assume that she doesn't like me unless she shows clear evidence to that effect. I will allow for the fact that she may like me a little or be neutral towards me.

11 If the woman at the party dislikes me and this is due to my having a dislikeable trait then this trait only proves that I am a fallible human being with a dislikeable trait. It doesn't mean that I am worthless.

11 When I conclude that I am not worthless if the woman at the party dislikes me, but that I am a fallible human being, then I am making a true statement.

12 If the woman at the party dislikes me, she may well be saying more about her preferences than about my worth. My worth can never be based on another person's preferences.

12 If the woman at the party dislikes me, and this is due to my having a dislikeable trait, then this trait only proves that I am a fallible human being with a dislikeable trait. It doesn't mean that I am worthless.

13 When I evaluate myself as worthless because the woman at the party dislikes me, then this is an arrant overgeneralization. In doing so, I am making the part–whole error even if I have a dislikeable trait. It is not sensible for me to rate my whole self on the basis of a part of me or on the basis of one of my experiences.

13 If the woman at the party dislikes me, she may well be saying more about her preferences than about me as a person. The fact that I am a fallible human being is true, no matter what her preferences are.

14 When I say that I am worthless if the woman at the party dislikes me, then I will be anxious when I am around her.

14 When I accept myself as a fallible human being in the face of the woman at the party disliking me, then this is a logical conclusion.

15 When I say that I am worthless when the woman at the party dislikes me, then I will be depressed for days afterwards.

15 When I say that I am a fallible human being if the woman at the party dislikes me, then I will be concerned, but not anxious, when I am around her, particularly as I want her to like me, but not insist that she does so.

16 When I conclude that I am worthless if the woman at the party dislikes me, then I will tend to think that it is a fact that she dislikes me in the absence of any evidence.

16 When I say that I am a fallible human being, worthless when the woman at the party dislikes me, then I will be sad, but not depressed, since I would like her to like me, but do not demand that she must.

17 When I conclude that I am worthless if the woman at the party dislikes me, then I will be sceptical of her friendliness towards me. I will tend to conclude that she is only being friendly towards me because she feels sorry for me or that she has an ulterior motive for being friendly.

17 When I conclude that I am a fallible human being if the woman at the party dislikes me, then I will tend not to conclude that she dislikes me in the absence of any evidence. I will take on board that she may have a range of responses towards me and will decide on her attitude towards me on the basis of evidence.

18 When I say that I am worthless if and when the woman at the party dislikes me, then I will tend to think that most other people will dislike me. How can anybody like a worthless person?

18 When I conclude that I am a fallible human being if the woman at the party dislikes me, then I will accept her friendliness towards me at face value. I will not think that she is bound to have an ulterior motive or that she feels sorry for me.

19 If I consider myself worthless if the woman at the party dislikes me, I will tend to avoid other social gatherings and will deprive myself of much pleasure.

19 When I say that I am a fallible human being if and when the woman at the party dislikes me, then I will not generalize from this event and think that most other people will also dislike me. I will judge each person's reaction towards me on evidence.

20 If the woman at the party clearly shows that she likes me, I may well wrongly tend to conclude that I am a worthwhile person. In doing so, I will reinforce my unhealthy belief that my worth is dependent on people liking me.

20 If I accept myself as a fallible human being if the woman at the party dislikes me, I will still attend other social gatherings and will experience the pleasure of doing so.

21 If the woman at the party clearly shows that she likes me, I will still consider myself to be the same fallible human being as I would be if she disliked me. I will not change my opinion of my self on the basis of people's attitude towards me.

Here are the instructions that I usually give people to help them to develop a rational portfolio.

1 Take one of your unhealthy beliefs and the healthy alternative to this belief. For your unhealthy belief include both your demand and self-depreciation statement and for your healthy belief include both the full preference and the self-acceptance statement.
2 Write each belief on a separate piece of paper under the appropriate heading as follows:

Unhealthy belief   *Healthy belief*

3 Take your unhealthy belief and write down as many persuasive arguments as you can think of against this unhealthy belief. If you get stuck remember that such beliefs are false, illogical and yield poor results.
4 Next, take your healthy belief and write down as many persuasive arguments as you can think of in support of this healthy belief. If you get stuck remember that such beliefs are true, logical and yield good results.
5 You may, if you so wish, do Step 4 before Step 3. Experiment to see which order you find most helpful.

Pitfalls in using the rational portfolio technique

In constructing a rational portfolio, it is important to guard against making incorrect arguments and irrelevant arguments. I will deal with each in turn.

Dealing with incorrect arguments

When you construct a rational portfolio you may make the following incorrect arguments: errors of fact, errors of logic and errors of helpfulness. Let me demonstrate what I mean by considering the following incorrect arguments that Liam, one of the 'Developing Self-acceptance' group members, put forward in his rational portfolio. Liam's unhealthy and healthy beliefs were as follows:

> *Unhealthy belief* My girlfriend must only be interested in me. If she is interested in another man it means that I am not good enough as a person.
>
> *Healthy belief* I want my girlfriend to be only interested in me, but she doesn't have to be. If she is interested in someone else it doesn't mean that I am not good enough as a person. I am a worthwhile person because I am human, alive and unique.

Errors of fact

When you make an error of fact in your rational portfolio you may come up with an argument showing why your unhealthy belief is false, which does not, in fact, do this, or you may put forward an argument showing why your healthy belief is true, which again fails to do so.

Thus, Liam developed the following argument purporting to show that his unhealthy belief was false: 'My girlfriend doesn't have to be only interested in me because I don't have to be only interested in her.'

Liam's argument is an error of fact for the following reason. By saying that she doesn't have to be only interested in him BECAUSE he believes that he doesn't have to be only interested in her, Liam is still implying that if he doesn't allow himself to be interested in another woman then his girlfriend must not be interested in another man. A factual argument would have been: 'Even if I am only interested in my girlfriend there is still no reason why she must only be interested in me.'

Errors of logic

When you make an error of logic in your rational portfolio you may come up with an argument showing why your unhealthy belief is illogical, which does not, in fact, do this, or you may put forward an argument showing why your healthy belief is logical, which again fails to do so.

Thus, Liam developed the following argument purporting to show that his unhealthy belief was illogical: 'I know that I am good enough as a person because other women find me attractive.'

Here Liam has shifted the goalposts and hasn't dealt with the conclusion that he wouldn't be good enough if his girlfriend were to be interested in other men. He could still believe that his worth goes down if this bad event happened because he is saying that his worth goes up if good events occur. Thus, he is still making the illogical error that his worth as a person depends on changing conditions. Instead, a better logical argument would be as follows: 'If my girlfriend was interested in another man that would be very bad, but it would not be logical to say that my worth would go down because of that bad event. My worth is fixed as long as I am alive, human and unique.'

Errors of helpfulness

When you make an error of helpfulness in your rational portfolio you may come up with an argument showing why your unhealthy belief is unhelpful, which does not, in fact, do this, or you may put forward an argument showing why your healthy belief is helpful, which again fails to do so.

For example, Liam developed the following argument to show why his healthy belief was helpful: 'Because I am worthwhile for being human, alive and unique, it doesn't matter if my girlfriend is interested in someone else.' The problem with this argument is that Liam is saying that it is helpful to feel indifferent if his girlfriend is interested in another man. But his healthy belief states that he would prefer it if his girlfriend was only interested in him even though he acknowledges that she doesn't have to be. Now, with that belief he would feel healthily disappointed or concerned if his girlfriend were interested in another man. To feel indifferent in these circumstances would involve Liam lying to himself, which is not a very helpful outcome for him.

Dealing with irrelevant arguments

Sometimes the arguments that you may employ in your rational portfolio may not be directed at your unhealthy or healthy belief at all. Thus, one of the arguments that Liam used to show that his unhealthy belief was false was as follows: 'I have no evidence that my girlfriend is interested in anyone else, so it's a good bet that she is only interested in me.' This argument is, in fact, directed at Liam's inference that his girlfriend is interested in someone else and is not an argument against his unhealthy belief: 'My girlfriend must only be interested in me. If she is interested in another man it means that I am not good enough as a person.' In fact, his argument does not have any bearing on this belief at all. Thus, when you are constructing arguments which either support your healthy belief or are against your unhealthy belief, make sure that these arguments are directed at your healthy and unhealthy beliefs and not at any other type of thought, like an inference. Thus, when checking your rational portfolio arguments ask yourself: 'Is my argument in favour of my healthy belief (i.e. full preference and self-acceptance belief) or against my unhealthy belief (i.e. demand and self-depreciation belief). If the answer is no, do not include the argument in your rational portfolio.

Make a point of carrying your rational portfolio around with you. This is helpful for two main reasons. First, if new arguments occur to you you can add them to your portfolio there and then. Second, taking your portfolio with you helps you to develop the habit of reviewing the arguments in your portfolio several times a day. So make regular reviews of your rational portfolio an important part of your journey toward greater self-acceptance.

The attack–response technique

A powerful way of strengthening your healthy beliefs is to attack them and respond effectively and persuasively to these attacks. A technique that capitalizes on this principle is known as the attack–response technique. Here is how to use this method.

1 Write down on a piece of paper the healthy belief that you wish to strengthen. I suggest that you include both your full preference and your self-acceptance belief. However, you can employ this technique with each component separately.
2 Rate your present level of conviction in this healthy belief on a 100-point scale, with 0 = no conviction and 100 = total conviction, and write down this rating below the healthy belief.
3 Attack this healthy belief as genuinely as you can. This attack will probably take the form of another unhealthy belief or a doubt, reservation or objection to the healthy belief. Write down this attack below the conviction rating.

4 Respond to this attack as fully as you can. It is really important that you respond to each element of this attack. Do so as persuasively as possible and write down this response below the attack.

5 Continue in this vein until you have made all your attacks and cannot think of any more.

If you find this exercise difficult, you might find it easier to make your attacks gently at first. Then, when you find that you can respond to these attacks quite easily, begin to make the attacks more biting. Work in this way until you are making really strong attacks. When you make an attack, do so as if you want yourself to believe it. Similarly, when you respond to your attacks, really throw yourself into it with the intention of demolishing the attack and raising your level of conviction in your healthy belief. Don't forget that the purpose of the exercise is to strengthen your healthy belief, so it is important that you stop when you have fully answered all of your attacks.

6 When you have responded to all of your attacks, write down your original healthy belief (i.e. the belief you wanted to strengthen) and then re-rate your level of conviction in it, using the same 100-point scale that you employed before. You will probably find that this rating has gone up. If it hasn't, look again at what you wrote and see if you can spot occasions when you didn't respond to an attack or to an element of an attack, or instances where your responses to attacks were not persuasive. In either case, re-do that part of the attack–response sequence until your new conviction rating has increased.

Let me now demonstrate how Mandy used the attack–response technique to good effect.

Healthy belief:	'I want to be able to impress my boss, but I don't have to do so. If I fail to impress him this does not mean that I am a failure, it means that I am a fallible human being who has failed in this respect.'
Conviction rating:	45%
Attack:	Yes, that's all very well, but your boss pays you very well and therefore is entitled to be impressed by your work. Since he pays you well, you have to impress him.
Response:	I do not deny that my boss pays me well, and he may be entitled to be impressed with me, although I am not quite sure what you mean by

the term 'entitled'. However, if there was a law of the universe decreeing that therefore I must impress him, then there is no way that I could fail to do so. But I am a human being, damn it, not a robot, and sometimes I may fail to do impressive work. Also, I may do impressive work and my boss may still not be impressed by it. I only have control over my behaviour, and not total control at that. I don't have control over his response to my behaviour.

Attack: But that's just an excuse for shoddy work. If you do shoddy work then you are a failure.

Response: Of course what I have just said is not an excuse for shoddy work. It is a full explanation for why I do not have to be able to impress my boss. Don't forget that if I give up my demand about being able to impress my boss, I still have my healthy desire to be able to do so, and that desire as well as my own standards for myself about doing well will motivate me to do the best that I can. Shoddy work is much more likely to stem from my being indifferent about being able to impress my boss than from my desire to be able to do so.

Second, you say that I would be a failure if I did shoddy work. Let me address that. To be a failure as a person means that I would have to fail at everything that I turned my hand to, now, in the past and in the future. That is completely ridiculous. There are lots of things that I do well, lots that I don't do well and lots that are average. That makes me a fallible human being, not a failure. You are making the mistake of rating me as a person on the basis of the quality of my work, but that is again ridiculous. First, I am far too complex to give myself a single rating, which is what being a failure means in this context, and second, doing so involves my making the part–whole error where I think that I can judge the whole of me by judging a part. If I do shoddy work that is just a part of me and is hardly a good guide to the rest of me. That's just like buying a house because you like the door knocker. Now if I am a fallible human being and not a failure for doing shoddy work, this argument also applies if I am not able to impress my boss.

Attack: OK. You may not be a failure for not being able to impress your boss, but surely you would be worthier if you did impress him than if you didn't.

Response: Nice try, but that argument won't wash either. By saying that I would be worthier if I were able to impress than if I were unable to do so is again assuming that you can rate me as a human being and that my worth varies according to the presence or absence of my ability to impress my boss. You can say with justification that being able to impress my boss is better than not being able to do so, but it is wholly illegitimate to go from there to conclude that my worth varies as a result.

Original healthy belief: 'I want to be able to impress my boss, but I don't have to do so. If I fail to impress him this does not mean that I am a failure, it means that I am a fallible human being who has failed in this respect.'

New conviction rating: 75%

There are two other variations of the attack–response technique that you might wish to use. The first involves your putting your attacks and responses on to audiotape so that when you replay the dialogue, you can evaluate not only the content of the arguments that you employed, but the tone in which you made them. It is important that the tone of your responses is more powerful and convincing than the tone of your attacks. If the reverse is the case then your conviction ratings in your healthy belief will not go up and may even go down. Thus, when you are using the tape-recorded version of the attack–response technique, try to make your responses sound more powerful and more persuasive than your attacks by modifying your tone of voice accordingly.

The second variation of attack–response that I wish to discuss is known as the devil's advocate technique. You need to ask a friend to help you by attacking your healthy belief. In particular, ask your friend to attack your healthy belief in the way that you did in the written and tape-recorded versions of this technique, while your task is to respond effectively and persuasively to his or her attacks. You may have to explain the nature of healthy and unhealthy beliefs (with special reference to demands and self-depreciation beliefs on the one hand and full preferences and self-acceptance beliefs on the other hand) to your friend before your friend is able to play the role of devil's advocate properly, but if done well this technique can help you to strengthen your healthy beliefs in a powerful way.

Should these three versions of the attack–response technique be done in any set order? The answer is no, but I tend to recommend that you do the written version first, before you tackle the tape-recorded version, while the devil's advocate version can best be employed last. I recommend this order because in my experience it best facilitates the development of competence in the use of the attack–response technique.

Pitfalls in using the attack–response technique and its variants

When you use the attack–response technique, it is important that you guard against making the following mistakes.

Failing to attack the healthy belief

When this happens it is likely to send you off track. For example, imagine that Mandy presented the following as an attack on her healthy belief:

Healthy belief:	'I want to be able to impress my boss, but I don't have to do so. If I fail to impress him this does not mean that I am a failure, it means that I am a fallible human being who has failed in this respect.'
Attack:	But if you don't impress your boss, this will mean that he won't like you.

This attack does not directly attack Mandy's rational belief. Rather, it puts forward an inferential connection between one inference ('I will not be able to impress my boss') and another ('My boss will not like me if I do not impress him'). It does not, in fact, put forward an attack on

Mandy's rational belief. A better attack would have been one directly at Mandy's healthy belief, such as:

'But your boss pays your wages, therefore you have to be able to impress him.'

Failing to respond to the attack

You may have successfully directed your attack to your healthy belief, but you not have responded effectively and persuasively to that attack.

Let's take the example of Carol. Her rational belief was as follows: 'I'd much rather I hadn't hurt my children's feelings but very unfortunately there's no reason why this absolutely should not have happened. I'm not a rotten person for hurting their feelings. I'm a fallible human being who did a very unfortunate thing.'

Carol's attack on this newly constructed healthy belief was as follows: 'Of course you're a bad person. If you weren't, you wouldn't have hurt their feelings.'

Carol then responded to this attack as follows: 'But I didn't mean to hurt their feelings. I love them really.' The difficulty with this response, as you can see, is that it does not actually respond to the attack, namely that Carol is a rotten person for hurting her children's feelings. It just makes the point that it was not her intention to hurt their feelings. A better targeted response would have been the one that Carol eventually developed: 'I'm not a bad person whether or not I meant to hurt my children's feelings. If I was a bad person, I could only do bad things and that is obviously ridiculous. No, even though I hurt their feelings, I'm not bad; I'm fallible and unrateable even though it is bad that my children's feelings may have been hurt.'

Failing to respond to all elements of an attack

Sometimes you may respond to some elements of an attack, but not all. Consequently, certain elements (including key elements) may be left unchallenged and may exert a deleterious effect on you. When this happens while using this technique, I suggest that you do the following. First, acknowledge and be pleased with the fact that you did respond accurately to certain elements of the attack. Then formulate a response which does deal accurately with the unchallenged elements of the attack, ensuring that you have put forward answers to each unchallenged element.

Let us see how this helped Lionel, whose healthy belief was as follows: 'I'd rather not play poorly in front of my golfing colleagues, but there is no law preventing me from doing so. If I play poorly, I'm not an insignificant person, but a fallible human being who can play well, poorly and averagely.'

Lionel's attack and immediate response to the attack was as follows:

Lionel's attack: But I am not supposed to play poorly. If I do so, it must prove that I am less worthy than if I were to play well.

Lionel's response: My worth does not depend on how I play. My ability to play golf is just one aspect of me, not the whole of me. I am a complex, unrateable person. I can rate my golfing play, but not my self.

On reading over his response, Lionel acknowledged that he had responded to most of the attack. But he also acknowledged that he had not responded to the element of the attack which said that he was not supposed to play poorly. Then Lionel disputed this belief, saying, 'There is no law of the universe which decrees that I'm supposed to play well. I am not a golfing machine. I am a human being. Even Nick Faldo has his off days.'

Failing to develop persuasive responses to the attacks

Here, you make a well-targeted response to an attack but you do not find the response very persuasive. If this happens, you can either change the wording of your response or you can add to your response to make your argument more persuasive.

For example, Betty's healthy belief was as follows: 'I prefer to sing well in public, but I don't have to do so. If I do sing poorly in public, I'm not a fool, I'm fallible.'

Betty then attacked this belief as follows: 'But you have had all that training. You must be able to sing well in public after that.'

When Betty responded to it – 'There is no such law. If there was, I couldn't sing poorly' – she was not at all persuaded by this argument. So she thought long and hard and came up with the following response, which she found much more persuasive: 'If there was a law which said that I must be able to sing well in public, then I'd be a singing machine. That's a ridiculous notion. I'm a fallible human being and, as such, there is always the possibility that I might not sing well when I give a public recital. I don't like that, but I do acknowledge that this possibility exists.'

To sum up the best way of getting the most out of the attack–response technique:

1 Make sure that you attack the healthy belief that you are attempting to strengthen. If you fail to do so, you will deprive yourself of the opportunity of developing persuasive arguments to counter your attacks.
2 Make sure that you respond to your attack as directly as you can. Failure to do so means that your attack will remain intact and will prevent you from strengthening your conviction in your healthy belief.
3 Make sure that you respond to all elements of your attack. Otherwise, the unresponded-to elements will remain intact, and again this will prevent you from strengthening your conviction in your healthy belief.
4 Finally, make sure that each response to your attack is as persuasive as possible. If not, you will tend to maintain your conviction in your unhealthy belief.

The use of forceful self-statements

Early on, when I outlined to you the process of belief change, I mentioned that it was important to use force and energy when working to integrate your healthy beliefs into your belief system. One way of doing this is to use forceful self-statements. Take one or more of your healthy beliefs, which may take the form of a full preference, a self-acceptance belief or a combination of the two. Read this out to yourself, first in a powerful, forceful manner and then in a weak, 'namby-pamby' manner. Then ask yourself which of the two versions you found more persuasive. In all probability it was the version you read in a forceful manner.

Once you have seen the value of a forceful self-statement designed to promote unconditional self-acceptance, you need to do the following. First, repeat the statement out loud forcefully a few times. Then, whisper the statement, retaining the same level of force and energy as you did when you spoke the statement out loud. Finally, rehearse the healthy belief silently, retaining the same level of force and energy as before.

I suggest that you silently but forcefully rehearse your self-acceptance statements several times a day, even if you are not depreciating yourself. Thus, Mandy silently and forcefully rehearsed the self-statements: 'I can accept myself as a fallible human being even if I can't impress my boss' and 'I don't have to impress my boss, although it would be nice if I did' several times a day.

Make sure that you guard against a number or errors when using this technique

1 Don't change a full preference to a partial preference.

Say 'I want to give a good talk, but I don't have to do so', rather than 'I want to give a good talk.' It is much easier to transform a partial preference into a demand than it is to transform a full preference into a demand.

2 Don't introduce a note of indifference into your self-statement.

Say 'I want to give a good talk, but I don't have to do so', rather than 'I want to give a good talk and it doesn't matter if I don't.' Trying to convince yourself that you don't care when you do will not work and will ultimately impede your progress towards self-acceptance.

3 Don't just assert who you are not. Affirm who you are as well as who you are not.

Don't just say 'I am not a failure if I don't give a good talk', say 'I am not a failure if I don't give a good talk, I am a fallible human being who failed this time.' If you just assert who you are not without affirming who you are, you may still implicitly be adhering to conditional self-rating. For example, when you say that you are not a failure if you don't give a good talk, you could still imply that you would be worthier if you gave a good talk than if you didn't.

4 Don't confuse a trait statement with a self-acceptance statement.

Don't say 'Although I acted unkindly to my wife the other day, I am basically a kind person' because kindness is a trait and is not equivalent to your self. Instead, say 'I am a fallible human being who unfortunately acted unkindly to my wife the other day.' In this statement you are explicitly accepting your self.

The emotive-imagery technique

Another way of strengthening your conviction in your healthy belief is known as the emotive-imagery technique. Here is how to use this technique:

1 Identify a situation where you depreciated yourself and focus on the aspect of this situation that you were most disturbed about. You will recall from Chapter 4 that this aspect is known as the critical A.

2 Close your eyes and vividly imagine this situation, and focus on the critical A.

3 Identify and get in touch with the unhealthy belief that you held about the critical A.

4 Really get in touch with the disturbed emotion that you felt in the situation and stay with this emotion briefly (choose one from the following: anxiety, depression, shame, guilt, unhealthy anger, unhealthy jealousy, unhealthy envy or hurt).

5 While still imagining the same situation and focusing on the same critical A, change your unhealthy belief to its healthy alternative and stay with this new belief until you experience a healthy negative emotion about the negative event at A (one of the following: concern, sadness, disappointment, remorse, healthy anger, healthy jealousy, healthy envy or sorrow).

6 Keep this healthy belief in mind and keep experiencing the associated healthy negative emotion for about five minutes, all the time imagining the situation you have previously identified, and in particular focusing on the critical A.

7 Practise this technique at least three times a day for five minutes each time.

In using the emotive-imagery technique, Mandy closed her eyes and imagined showing her boss a piece of work that she thought a lot of and him saying that the work was OK, but could be a lot better. In doing so, Mandy focused on her seeming inability to impress her boss. As she did so, Mandy rehearsed her unhealthy belief: 'I must be able to impress my boss, and if I can't I am a failure', and got in touch briefly with her feelings of depression. Then Mandy changed her belief to: 'I'd prefer to be able to impress my boss, but I don't have to do so. I am not a failure if I can't impress him. I am a fallible human being whether I impress my boss or not', while focusing on not being able to impress her boss and feeling sad, but not depressed, about this. Mandy maintained her healthy belief in this scene and focused on her healthy sadness for five minutes. Mandy practised the emotive-imagery technique three times a day for five minutes each time.

As you practise the emotive-imagery technique, it is important to bear in mind the following points:

• Select a specific event to imagine, not a generalized event.

• Focus on the aspect of the event that you particularly put yourself down about. Don't just imagine the event as such, but zero in on the bit that you found most painful.

- Keep imagining that most painful aspect of the event while rehearsing your unhealthy belief.
- Identify and experience your one predominant unhealthy negative emotion. You may have experienced more than one emotion, but get in touch with the emotion about the critical A.
- As you change your unhealthy belief to its healthy alternative, make sure that you keep focusing on the critical A.
- As you focus on your new healthy negative emotion, make it the same intensity as your unhealthy negative emotion. It is not necessarily healthy for you to experience a mild emotion about a really aversive activating event.
- As you practise this technique, spend much more time imagining yourself dealing with the event in a self-accepting way than in a self-depreciating way.
- After a while you can just imagine the negative event and in particular the critical aspect of that event; rehearse your healthy belief and experience the associated healthy negative emotion.
- Practise this technique at odd moments of the day when you have a small amount of time on your hands. Practise it while waiting for a bus, for example, or riding on the Underground. After all, you have probably gained a lot of mental practice rehearsing your unhealthy self-depreciating beliefs and associated demands in a variety of negative life events, so you do need a lot of corrective practice of rehearsing your healthy full preferences and self-acceptance beliefs.

In this chapter, I have introduced a number of techniques which you can use to strengthen your conviction in the beliefs that make up a philosophy of unconditional self-acceptance. Regular practice of these techniques is needed if you are to proceed along the road to self-acceptance. However, unless you act in ways that are consistent with your self-acceptance beliefs and associated full preferences, you will not progress far along this road, for taking appropriate action in the world is also an important ingredient in the development of self-acceptance, as I will explain in the following chapter.

7

Act on Your Healthy Beliefs

In the previous chapter, I described a number of thinking-based techniques that have been devised to help you to strengthen your conviction in the beliefs that underpin a philosophy of unconditional self-acceptance and to weaken your conviction in the beliefs that lie at the root of self-depreciation or low self-esteem. I mentioned at the end of that chapter that taking appropriate action is also an important ingredient in the development of self-acceptance. In fact, the more I work in the field of counselling and the more I endeavour to help my clients develop unconditional self-acceptance, the more I see how crucial such action is in the change process.

I feel so strongly about this point that you may find what I have to say on the subject somewhat repetitive. I don't apologize for this because I want to make sure that I get across the following two points:

1 One of the best ways of developing self-acceptance is to practise thinking self-accepting ideas AND TO ACT IN WAYS THAT ARE CONSISTENT WITH THESE IDEAS.
2 If you practise thinking self-accepting ideas, but act in ways that are inconsistent with these ideas and are, in fact, consistent with self-depreciation ideas, then you will be more convinced by your actions than by your thoughts.

Let me offer you two formulas that make these points in ways that might help you remember them:

- SELF-ACCEPTANCE THINKING + ACTION BASED ON SELF-ACCEPTANCE = INCREASED CONVICTION IN YOUR SELF-ACCEPTANCE PHILOSOPHY

- SELF-ACCEPTANCE THINKING + ACTION BASED ON SELF-DEPRECIATION = DECREASED CONVICTION IN YOUR SELF-ACCEPTANCE PHILOSOPHY

If you find these formulas helpful, write them down on a 5×3 card and review it several times a day.

Let me illustrate this phenomenon by an example. Henrietta was working to give up her dire need for approval and to accept herself in the face of disapproval. She had employed all the techniques that I have presented in the previous two chapters and was ready to put her gains into practice behaviourally with someone she was sure disapproved of her whom she had previously studiously avoided. Henrietta arranged to meet with the woman who, sure enough, showed clearly that she disapproved of Henrietta. Henrietta duly practised the idea that she didn't need this woman's approval and that she could accept herself even though the woman disliked her. However, almost in the same breath, the woman asked Henrietta to do something that was clearly unreasonable and Henrietta agreed. Later, Henrietta realized that she had acceded to the woman's unreasonable request because she believed that she had to have the woman's approval.

Using the framework that I have introduced to you, let us examine Henrietta's options and consider the effects of each.

Option 1:   Henrietta could have avoided seeing the woman and not rehearsed her self-acceptance belief.

This is probably one of the two worst options on offer because Henrietta is neither practising her healthy belief, nor acting in a way that clearly strengthens her unhealthy belief. Since she believes that she must not be disapproved by the woman in question, an efficient way of avoiding disapproval from the woman is to avoid her altogether. However, this action, while protecting Henrietta in the short term, only serves to perpetuate her self-depreciating belief in the longer term.

Option 2:   Henrietta could have seen the woman, not rehearsed her self-acceptance belief and agreed to the woman's unreasonable request.

This is another poor option for Henrietta's prospects for developing self-acceptance. While in this scenario Henrietta is not avoiding the woman, which is good, it is very likely that by not rehearsing her self-acceptance belief she will, in fact, be implicitly rehearsing her self-depreciation belief. In addition, by acceding to the woman's unreasonable request, Henrietta is, in fact, acting in a way that is consistent with this self-depreciation idea.

Option 3:   Henrietta could have seen the woman, rehearsed her self-acceptance belief and agreed to the woman's unreasonable request.

This is the option that Henrietta did choose and, as I have already discussed, the problem with this option is that Henrietta is undermining the work that she is doing in her head to develop a philosophy of unconditional self-acceptance by acting against this idea in practice. The fact that she did agree to do the task in question was, as Henrietta saw later, based on the opposite idea that she did need the other woman's approval. Why else, she acknowledged, would she have done the task, which was quite unreasonable, if she did not believe that she had to turn the woman's disapproval into approval?

Option 4: Henrietta could have seen the woman, not practised her self-accepting belief and refused the woman's unreasonable request.

In this scenario Henrietta is acting healthily by seeing the woman in the first place and by refusing to accede to her unreasonable request in the second. However, because she is not rehearsing her self-acceptance belief we are not sure (and neither can Henrietta be sure) that her actions will lead to increased self-acceptance. For example, Henrietta might conclude on the basis of her behaviour that she is superior to the woman concerned, or if nothing untoward happened she might conclude that she was wrong about the woman, who wasn't as critical as she had thought. What she hasn't done, however, is to practise accepting herself in the face of possible rejection from the woman.

As I tell my clients, healthy behaviour will help to change your thinking, but on its own, without concomitant rehearsal of healthy beliefs, there is no way of knowing how your thinking will change, whereas healthy behaviour and concomitant rehearsal of healthy beliefs will help you to increase your conviction in these beliefs.

Option 5: Henrietta could have seen the woman, practised her self-accepting ideas and refused the woman's unreasonable request.

This is the best option of all, because everything is consistent and in the direction of self-acceptance. First, Henrietta is confronting the woman; second, she is practising her self-accepting belief; and third, by refusing to comply with the woman's unreasonable request, Henrietta is acting in a way that is consistent with her self-acceptance idea. She is telling herself that she does not need the woman's approval and she is acting as if she does not need her approval.

I hope now that you can see clearly that the best way to further your path towards greater self-acceptance is by rehearsing the full preferences and self-acceptance ideas that comprise your self-acceptance philosophy and by acting in ways that are consistent with these beliefs.

So go back to your list of problems and goals that you developed in Chapter 3 and, taking them one at a time, resolve to follow the constructive forms of behaviour that you outlined there. Make a sensible plan to confront situations that are important to face if you are to progress along the path towards self-acceptance. If need be, rank these situations according to how difficult you would find it to face them and work your way up this hierarchy, facing these situations while strongly rehearsing your self-acceptance ideas at the same time. Resist any urges to go back to your more ingrained, more familiar, but ultimately self-defeating behaviour. Familiarize yourself with your self-defeating behaviours as you listed them in Chapter 3, and be on guard against 'mindlessly' slipping back into these old ways of behaving. It is very easy for you to return to patterns of behaviour that are consistent with the self-depreciation beliefs that you are trying to surrender, but which give you short-term relief when you are uncomfortable. Tolerate this discomfort and show yourself strongly that it is worth tolerating this discomfort, because doing so will help you stay on the path towards self-acceptance. If you have particular trouble dealing with discomfort in this way, you might find it helpful to consult the book that I wrote with my colleague, Jack Gordon, entitled *Beating the Comfort Trap* (Sheldon Press, 1993).

In the same regard, remind yourself from the work you did on the issue in Chapter 3 of how you have acted in the past to compensate for your self-depreciation problem and what you can do instead that is both constructive and non-compensating. Resolve to act in these constructive ways whenever you feel the urge to compensate for your self-depreciation and rehearse your self-acceptance ideas at the same time.

In short, while being sensible and non-perfectionistic, make use of and seek out opportunities to practise your self-accepting philosophy and to act in ways that are consistent with this philosophy whenever it is feasible for you to do so. If you work in this way through your problem list and towards your goals you will help yourself move from intellectual insight into a philosophy of unconditional self-acceptance to greater emotional insight into this philosophy, where you integrate this philosophy into your belief system so that it has significant impact on how you feel, think and behave.

The use of mental rehearsal

Once you have decided to practise acting in a way that is consistent with your developing self-acceptance beliefs and associated full preferences, you might find it helpful to rehearse what you are going to do before you do it. Mental rehearsal can be a very powerful technique for some but unhelpful for others, so I suggest that you try it to determine how helpful it will be for you as a preparation for action in the real world.

It can be useful to practise imagining carrying out behaviour both where you encounter a negative activating event and where you encounter a positive activating event. In doing so you will prepare yourself for the worst and you will also realize that a good outcome is possible. Let me illustrate how to use mental rehearsal by showing how I encouraged Sarah to use it. Sarah's chosen task was to speak up at two seminars and to practise showing herself that she is not a stupid person if she says something stupid. Rather, she is an unrateable person who acted stupidly on one occasion. I begin the interchange:

Windy:	Sarah, close your eyes and imagine that you are in your seminar group and see yourself saying something stupid. When you have done so, rehearse in your mind the statement, 'I am not a stupid person for saying something stupid. I am an unrateable person who said something stupid on this occasion.' Can you see yourself doing this?
Sarah (after 30 seconds):	Yes, I can.
Windy:	Now how do feel when you say this to yourself?
Sarah:	Disappointed that I said something stupid.
Windy:	But not ashamed?
Sarah:	No.
Windy:	Good. Now the next step is for you to practise seeing yourself speaking and not saying something stupid. This is important, because it is also possible that what you say will make sense. It's important that you prepare yourself for both a bad outcome and a good outcome. So close your eyes and imagine that you are speaking in your seminar group while rehearsing your self-acceptance belief. Can you see yourself doing this?

Sarah (after 35 seconds):	Yes, I can.
Windy:	And how do you feel seeing yourself do this?
Sarah:	Pleased.
Windy:	Excellent. So before you actually go to your next seminar group and practise this in real life, I suggest that you practise these imagery exercises two or three times a day. Start off imagining the worst and then practise seeing a favourable outcome in your mind's eye.

Here are the steps that you need to follow when practising mental rehearsal of thinking-behavioural tasks:

1 Select a task that you have decided to carry out in the service of self-acceptance.
2 Close your eyes and picture yourself doing the task and practising your self-acceptance belief while facing a negative outcome. Experience the healthy negative emotion that stems from the healthy belief.
3 Then, practise seeing yourself doing the task and practising your self-acceptance belief while facing a positive outcome. Experience pleasure at this outcome.
4 Practise mental rehearsal of both these scenarios two or three times a day before you do the thinking-behavioural task in real life.

The issue of self-confidence

A lot of people say that they lack self-confidence and want to become more self-confident. At first glance there seems nothing wrong with this as a goal, but if we take a closer look at the concept of self-confidence, problems begin to appear – similar problems, in fact, to those that exist with the concept of self-esteem. Let's examine the concept of self-confidence more closely. It is made up of two parts: 'self' and 'confidence'. As we have already seen, the term 'self' refers to everything about you that can be rated. The term 'confidence' means having faith or trust that you can do something. So self-confidence means having faith and trust that you can do everything that relates to your 'self'. Obviously this is a tall order and, for this reason and for the fact that self-confidence seems to imply self-rating, in Rational Emotive

Behaviour Therapy we discourage people from striving for self-confidence. Instead we encourage people to strive for greater task confidence based on a healthy philosophy of unconditional self-acceptance. Task confidence means faith or trust that you can do a particular task.

Now, if you wish to become proficient at something which you value and which you are not very good at or which you are approaching for the first time, you will not be confident at it. Since you have little or no success experience at the task in question you can hardly have faith that you can do it. You only develop task confidence when you achieve a number of such successes, and this means two things: learning how to do the task, and doing the task UNCONFIDENTLY at first until you begin to become confident at it. When you do something unconfidently at first the chances are that you will do it poorly. This is where accepting yourself is so important. If you accept yourself for your initial failures then you are more likely to learn from your failures, and hence more likely to persist at the task than if you were to depreciate yourself instead.

I hope you can see that striving for task confidence based on unconditional self-acceptance is more realistic, more logical and more likely to be achieved than striving for self-confidence, with its emphasis on having faith that you can do virtually everything that you turn your hand to.

If you want to do something that you prize, recognize that you will not be confident at it at first. So do it unconfidently and accept yourself for, and learn from, the mistakes that you invariably will make. Persist in this way until you become confident and competent at the task in question. In short, proceed on the principle of task confidence based on self-acceptance rather than on the principle of self-confidence.

Shame-attacking exercises

So far the work you have done to help yourself along the road to self-acceptance has been serious. Now is the time to have a bit of fun along this road. Shame-attacking exercises involve you acting 'shamefully' in public and practising self-acceptance beliefs as you do so. It is important for you to do shame-attacking exercises for the following reasons:

1 Shame involves self-depreciation. Consequently, 'attacking' your shame helps you to develop a philosophy of unconditional self-acceptance.

2 You often limit yourself significantly because you are scared of what

others think of you. Doing shame-attacking exercises helps you to accept yourself in the face of public disapproval.

3 Consequently, in devising shame-attacking exercises, it is important to plan to do something that will attract the attention and disapproval of others.

4 When you do a shame-attacking exercise, remain in the situation and maintain eye contact. Leaving the situation immediately after you have done a shame-attacking exercise or avoiding eye contact with those present are two ways of helping you to feel better in the short term, but prevent you from accepting yourself in the situation concerned.

5 Take suitable action to protect yourself and others from harm. Thus, when devising a shame-attacking exercise make sure that you do not do anything that will:

- alarm others;
- offend your and others' moral codes;
- break the law;
- jeopardize your job or your friendships.

6 Develop and practise healthy self-acceptance beliefs and high frustration tolerance (HFT) beliefs before you do the task, while doing it and after you have done the exercise.

7 Use the emotive-imagery technique (see Chapter 6) before you carry out your shame-attacking exercise.

8 Identify and overcome blocks to carrying out your shame-attacking exercises.

Here are a few examples of shame-attacking exercises:

- wearing different coloured shoes;
- asking to buy a three-piece suite in a sweet shop;
- singing off-key in public;
- asking for directions to a town one is already in;
- shouting out the stops on a train;
- shouting out the time in a department store.

What are the ingredients of a good shame-attacking exercise? I would say that if you do the assignment, receive social disapproval which you fully focus on and practise accepting yourself in the face of such disapproval, then the presence of these three ingredients constitutes a shame-attacking exercise that has therapeutic value. While you may be relieved if nobody notices your 'shameful' behaviour or if nobody shows you disapproval, these conditions will not help you in the long run. So if this happens to you, continue to do shame-attacking exercises until people notice AND disapprove of you.

Finally, you will find doing shame-attacking exercises uncomfortable and in some cases very uncomfortable. As such, it is also helpful to tell yourself that you can stand the discomfort of doing these exercises, and that it is worth tolerating the discomfort of doing them because they have the potential of helping you further along the road towards unconditional self-acceptance.

Overcoming blocks to acting on your self-acceptance beliefs

As I have stressed throughout this chapter, acting in ways which are consistent with your developing self-acceptance beliefs and associated full preferences, and which in turn are inconsistent with your well-ingrained self-depreciation beliefs and associated demands is a powerful means of strengthening your conviction in your healthy beliefs. Put quite simply, unless you act on your healthy beliefs you will not proceed too far along the road towards self-acceptance.

While there are many obstacles to acting on your healthy beliefs that you may erect, in this chapter I will concentrate on three. These three obstacles can be summed up in the following three phrases:

- I must be confident before I act.
- I must have the courage to act before I act.
- I must be comfortable before I act.

If you hold any of these beliefs, then you will not act in ways that are consistent with your developing self-acceptance beliefs and related full preferences because you will tend not to be confident, feel courageous or feel comfortable taking this action. So in order to take the appropriate action, you need to challenge the above beliefs using the methods I have described in Chapters 5 and 6. Your goal then is to work towards achieving the following healthy beliefs:

1 I'd like to be confident before I act, but I do not need to be. I can act even though I don't feel confident doing so, and in fact the only way I can develop confidence is by acting unconfidently. I resolve to do this.

2 I'd like to have the courage to act before I act, but I don't need to have

it. I can act even though I don't feel courageous, and in fact the only way I can develop courage is to do what I have decided to do uncourageously. I resolve to do this.

3 I'd like to be comfortable before I act, but I don't have to be. I can act even though I don't feel comfortable, and in fact the only way that I can be comfortable acting in the way that I have chosen to act is to do so uncomfortably. I resolve to do so.

With these healthy beliefs you will overcome the obstacles to acting in ways that are consistent with your self-acceptance beliefs and related full preferences. If you resolve to take such action regularly you will take important strides towards developing unconditional self-acceptance.

8

Develop a Realistic View of Yourself and Your Life Experiences

So far in this book, I have shown you that at the root of your problems with low self-esteem (or self-depreciation) lie a set of rigid demands and self-depreciation beliefs. I have stressed that if you wish to develop self-acceptance you need to challenge and change these rigid demands and self-depreciation beliefs and bed down, strengthen and act on an alternative set of full preferences and self-acceptance beliefs. In this chapter, I will show how your rigid demands lead you to think unrealistically about yourself and your life experiences, and what you need to do to think more realistically in these two areas.

In Chapter 2, I pointed out that when you hold a set of rigid demands and self-depreciation beliefs this affects the way that you feel and the way that you act. More specifically, when you hold such beliefs you are very likely to experience one or more unhealthy negative emotions (e.g. depression, anxiety, guilt, hurt, shame, unhealthy ego-defensive anger, unhealthy jealousy and unhealthy envy) and act (or 'feel' like acting) in one or more dysfunctional ways. In addition, when you hold a set of rigid demands and self-depreciation beliefs it is likely that your subsequent thinking about yourself and your life experiences is likely to be negatively distorted and unrealistic.

Beliefs affect subsequent thinking

Consider the case of Brian. Brian felt ashamed about being unassertive and avoided other people when he thought that he had revealed this weakness in public, because he believed that he must not have such a weakness and that he was a weak, defective person for being unassertive. Putting this into the ABC framework, we have:

A = My unassertiveness is a weakness.

B = 1) I must not have this weakness.
    2) I am a weak, defective person for being unassertive.

C (emotional) =   Shame
  (behavioural) =   Withdrawing from others when I think that I have revealed this weakness in public

In addition, Brian's rigid demand and self-depreciation belief about his unassertiveness led him to the unrealistic thought that if he shows that he is acting weakly by not asserting himself, other people will look down on him and take advantage of him. This example shows that Brian's unhealthy belief led not only to an unhealthy emotional consequence and a dysfunctional behavioural consequence, but also to an unrealistic thinking consequence, in this case the thought that people will look down on him and take advantage of him. Using the ABC framework we have:

A = My unassertiveness is a weakness.

B = 1) I must not have this weakness.
　　2) I am a weak, defective person for being unassertive.

C (thinking) = People will look down on me and take advantage of me.

What would happen to Brian's subsequent thinking if his beliefs were healthy? Let's see:

A = My unassertiveness is a weakness.

B = 1) I'd prefer not to have this weakness, but there is no reason why I must not have it.
　　2) I am not a weak, defective person for being unassertive. Rather, I am a fallible human being with weaknesses and strengths.

C (thinking) = People will have a range of responses towards me. Some may look down on me and take advantage of me, while others will show compassion towards me and be on my side.

As can be seen, Brian's healthy beliefs (at B) would have led him to think in a more realistic and balanced way (at C).

Thinking errors stem largely from unhealthy beliefs

Brian's example clearly shows that rigid demands and self-depreciation beliefs lead to thinking which is overly skewed to the negative, while full preferences and self-acceptance beliefs lead to thinking which is balanced and more realistic.

Thinking which stems from rigid demands and self-depreciation beliefs tends to be characterized by the following errors:

1 Overgeneralization – here you view a single, usually negative, event as a definite pattern (e.g. 'Because I made a grave error at the interview which proves that I am a fool, I will continue to make grave errors at interviews').

2 Focusing on the negative – where you edit out the positive features of a situation and concentrate on the negative features ('My tutor thought that my essay was moderately good, but it absolutely should have been very good. As I look at it again I can only see the essay's bad points').

3 Disqualifying the positive – where you are unable to accept positive feedback (e.g. compliments: 'My friend told me that she liked the way I looked, but since I think I am worthless for not being as attractive as I absolutely should be, I thought she was only saying this to be kind, and deep down she didn't mean it').

4 Black-and-white thinking – where you see things as being all good or all bad (e.g. 'I just failed my oral examination as I absolutely should not have done. I think it was a complete failure').

5 Mind reading – where you are convinced that others have a negative view of you (e.g. 'I disclosed a weakness in public which proves that I am inadequate, and I am sure that other people think of me as an idiot').

6 Always-and-never thinking – where you think that bad events will always occur and that good events will never occur (e.g. 'I failed my driving test, which I absolutely should have passed. This means that I will never pass it').

7 Minimization – where you play down your own achievements (e.g. 'I must do much better than other people. I did well on the task, but anybody could have done the task well').

8 Magnification – where you make more than is warranted of your failures (e.g. 'I fluffed my lines at the rehearsal, which proves that I am a worthless idiot. Nobody will forget what I did for a very long time').

9 Personalizing – where you think that you are the cause of something that was outside your control or where you think that others' responses are directed at you where corroborative evidence is not available (e.g. 'I played poorly at the match yesterday, which I absolutely should not have done. A group of people were laughing when I walked past and I am sure that they were laughing at me').

10 Negative prediction – where you predict negative events (e.g. 'I am a bad person for not visiting my parents and thus God will soon punish me').

11 Emotional reasoning – thinking that something is true because you

feel strongly that it is true (e.g. 'I am worthless and feel strongly that others think so too. My strong feelings about this prove that I am right').

12 Cognitive reasoning – thinking that your thoughts are inevitably a true guide to reality (e.g. 'I must know that people like me. If I think that someone dislikes me, this is proof that it is true').

As can be seen from the above, all of these thinking errors are produced not by the existence of negative events, but by the unhealthy beliefs the people concerned held about these events.

Thinking consequences can become inferences at A

The next point is important. Having created the thinking consequence of (in this case) an unhealthy belief, the person can then focus on this thinking consequence, which becomes a new activating event at A. The person can then hold a healthy or an unhealthy belief (at B) about this new A, which can then lead to a further set of emotional, behavioural and thinking consequences at C. In Brian's case (see above), when he held a set of unhealthy beliefs about his weakness (i.e. being assertive) he constructed a scenario in his mind (his thinking consequence) which was skewed to the negative (i.e. 'People will look down on me and take advantage of me'). He then focused on this consequence (which becomes his new A) and believed that this would prove that he was worthless. In this way, you may deepen your self-depreciating belief system.

You bring your tendencies to think unhealthily at B to your inferences at A, which are thus coloured by this unhealthy thinking

In the above section, I showed how unhealthy beliefs (at B in the ABC framework) lead to subsequent unrealistic thinking about oneself and one's life experiences (at C in the ABC framework). This unrealistic thinking often takes the form of negative distorted inferences, and when you focus on one of these inferences it serves as the A in the subsequent ABC episode.

In addition, it also happens that you bring your tendency to hold unhealthy beliefs to the events that you focus on in the first place (at A) and that these unhealthy beliefs lead you to make distorted inferences about these aspects. Thus, Brian brought his tendency to condemn himself for having weaknesses to the situation where he failed to assert himself, and this tendency influenced him to make the inference at A that lack of assertion is a weakness. When Brian accepted himself more for having weaknesses he came to see that lack of assertion was a reflection of an anxiety problem and was not a weakness.

As I have just demonstrated, once you have made some progress at accepting yourself, you will find it easier to think realistically at C in the ABC framework and you will bring your developing tendency to accept yourself to the events in your life at A, about which you will make more realistic inferences.

How to challenge unrealistic thinking about yourself and your life experiences

The best time to challenge your unrealistic thinking about yourself and your experiences is, as I have shown above, after you have made some progress at challenging your rigid demands and self-depreciation beliefs and have made corresponding progress at strengthening your alternative full preferences and self-acceptance beliefs. If you try to challenge this unrealistic thinking before you have challenged your unhealthy beliefs, any change you make in your thinking will be short-lived, because this unrealistic thinking stems largely from your unchallenged unhealthy beliefs.

How do you know that your thinking is unrealistic? By examining it and realizing that it contains one or more of the thinking errors that I discussed earlier in this chapter. Once you have decided that your thinking about yourself and your life experiences is unrealistic, how can you challenge it? By taking the following steps:

- Make sure that you have made some progress in changing your unhealthy belief to its healthy alternative at B so that you can adopt an objective standpoint when checking the validity of the thought that you consider may be unrealistic.
- Write down the thought you are checking on a piece of paper.
- Understand the possible distorting effect of your unhealthy belief on this thought.
- Look for evidence that supports and evidence that contradicts your thought and write this down under separate headings.
- Evaluate this evidence.
- Stand back and evaluate all the available information and select the most realistic thought.

Let me illustrate how Liam, one of my 'Developing Self-acceptance' group members, used these steps.

1 Make sure that you have made some progress in changing your unhealthy belief to its healthy alternative at B so that you can adopt an objective standpoint when checking the validity of the thought that you consider may be unrealistic

Liam had made some progress at challenging his unhealthy belief, 'My girlfriend must only be interested in me and if she is interested in someone else it means that I am not good enough as a person', and now believed more strongly his healthy belief, 'I'd prefer it if my girlfriend was only interested in me, but this isn't essential. If she is interested in another man, it does not mean that I am not good enough as a person. Rather, I am a worthwhile person whether or not she is interested in another man.'

2 Write down the thought you are checking on a piece of paper

Liam wrote down the thought 'When my girlfriend spoke to another man yesterday, it meant that she was interested in having a relationship with him.'

3 Understand the possible distorting effect of your unhealthy belief on this thought

Liam readily understood that his unhealthy belief, 'My girlfriend must only be interested in me and if she is interested in someone else it means that I am not good enough as a person', influenced him to make the inference that because his girlfriend spoke to another man yesterday she was interested in having a relationship with him.

4 Look for evidence that supports and evidence that contradicts your thought and write this down under separate headings

It is helpful to do these tasks separately, as Liam did:

Evidence that supports the inference that when my girlfriend spoke to another man yesterday it meant that she was interested in having a relationship with him:

- The fact that I was jealous meant that my girlfriend was interested in having a relationship with the man.
- She was laughing and joking with him.
- I thought she was having a relationship with him.

Evidence that contradicts or does not support the inference that when my girlfriend spoke to another man yesterday it meant that she was interested in having a relationship with him:

- She is naturally friendly and was just being friendly with the man.
- I've thought that she was interested in having a relationship with men that she has spoken to before, but as far as I am aware she never has.
- She may have found the man attractive, but that does not mean that she is interested in having a relationship with him. I find a lot of women attractive, but I'm not interested in having a relationship with any of them.
- She assures me that she is only interested in me.

5 Evaluate this evidence

Evaluating the supportive evidence

The fact that I was jealous meant that she was interested in having a relationship with the man.

This is emotional reasoning. My feeling of jealousy only proves that I am jealous and does not say anything about my girlfriend's interest or lack of interest in the man.

She was laughing and joking with him.

This could mean that she was interested in having a relationship with the man, but it could also mean that she was being friendly. My girlfriend is a friendly person and laughs and jokes with all kinds of people, including old men, women and children. This obviously doesn't mean that she wants to have a sexual or emotional relationship with them.

I thought she was having a relationship with him.

This is an example of cognitive reasoning – because I think something, it must be so. My thoughts are hunches about reality and may not be a good guide to reality.

Evaluating the contradictory evidence

She is naturally friendly and was just being friendly with the man.

This is probably the case, but I don't know for certain. This latter point is quite revealing, since I tend to think that not being certain that she isn't interested in having a relationship with someone means that she is interested. I tend to demand certainty and find it difficult to accept probability when it comes to my girlfriend.

I've thought that she was interested in having a relationship with men that she has spoken to before, but as far as I am aware she never has.

Again, as I believe that I can't stand uncertainty, I tend to think that not knowing for sure that my girlfriend hasn't had a relationship with someone means that she has. This just shows that I need to learn to go with probability and give up my demand for certainty.

She may have found the man attractive, but that does not mean that she is interested in having a relationship with him. I find a lot of women attractive, but I'm not interested in having a relationship with any of them.

This is true, although I also demand that she must only find me attractive. This is a double standard since I don't have this rule for myself.

She assures me that she is only interested in me.

My girlfriend is very honest and I'm pretty sure that if she was interested in the man she would tell me. She wouldn't lie, although I can't be 100 per cent certain of this. There I go again, demanding absolute certainty!

6 Stand back and evaluate all the available information and select the most realistic thought

Here, it is useful to ask yourself what conclusion an objective jury would come to when faced with the available evidence. Either accept or reject your original thought, and if you reject it settle on a thought which best fits the available evidence. This is what Liam did. His conclusion was as follows:

From what I have written it is clear to me that I am bringing a number of unhealthy beliefs to this situation and situations like it. My girlfriend is friendly and when she talks to people she laughs and jokes with them. She is also honest. I tend to be jealous and think that what I think and feel is a good indication of what is real, when objectively it isn't. I also see now that I demand certainty that my girlfriend isn't interested in men and think that lack of such certainty means that she definitely is interested in them.

Given all this information, I conclude that my girlfriend wasn't interested in having a relationship with the man in question. She was just being friendly with him. I will remember this the next time I think she is interested in having a relationship with someone else.

So far I have discussed and illustrated a procedure for challenging unrealistic thinking. This procedure is rather lengthy and there will be times when you need quicker ways of challenging unrealistic thoughts. What follows is a list of questions you can use to question thoughts which may be unrealistic. I suggest that you become familiar with the six-step procedure I outlined above before you use one or more of the following illustrative questions for challenging thoughts. Then use these questions when time is at a premium:

- What evidence do I have for this thought? Are there other ways of looking at the situation?
- How would someone else think about the situation?
- Am I forgetting relevant facts or overemphasizing irrelevant ones?
- Am I overestimating how likely this event is?
- How would an objective jury think about this situation?
- Would I urge a good friend to come to the same conclusion? If not, how would I advise him/her to think about the situation?
- How would I view this situation if I accepted myself?
- How would I view this situation if I held a full preference about it and not a rigid demand?
- Is it helpful for me to think this way? If not, what would be a more helpful way to view the situation?
- Is my thought true? If not, which thought would be true?
- Is my thought sensible/logical? If not, which way of thinking would be sensible/logical?
- Am I making a thinking error? If so, how would I think if I did not make this error?

When you ask yourself and answer these questions, do so first in writing until you become proficient at challenging your unrealistic thoughts. Then you will be more able to carry out this procedure in your head.

The strengths and weaknesses exercise

Why have I left it so long before encouraging you to list your strengths and weaknesses? You probably expected that I might start the book with this exercise. The reason I have left this task virtually until the end is that it is only now that you are most likely to benefit from it. Let me show you what I mean by asking you to list your strengths and weaknesses under two different sets of conditions: when you are depreciating yourself and when you are accepting yourself.

Condition 1: Strengths and weaknesses from the position of self-depreciation

First, get yourself into a self-depreciating state of mind. If you find this difficult (which actually is a good sign), review in your mind past situations where you put yourself down and strongly rehearse a self-depreciation belief until you feel badly about yourself. Then, while you are in this frame of mind, make two lists, one which lists your strengths as you see them and the other which lists your weaknesses as you see them.

Condition 2: Strengths and weaknesses from the position of self-acceptance

Now, get yourself into a self-accepting state of mind. Rehearse some of the full preferences and self-acceptance beliefs that you have been working on so far, and when you have done this again make two lists, one which lists your strengths as you see them and the other which lists your weaknesses as you see them.

What you will probably find is that when you are in a self-depreciating frame of mind, your list of weaknesses will be longer, perhaps even much longer, than your strengths. However, when you are in a self-accepting frame of mind, your two lists will be more equal in number. Also, your perceived weaknesses will be more realistic and less extreme in the self-acceptance condition than in the self-depreciation condition.

This exercise is designed primarily to show you two things. First, it demonstrates how your beliefs can affect your view of yourself, and second, it clearly indicates that the best time for you to review your strengths and weaknesses objectively is when you are in a self-accepting frame of mind. Once you are in a self-accepting state then you have the clarity of mind to decide which weaknesses you wish to focus on and change and how to go about doing this. You also have the clarity of mind to decide which strengths you wish to capitalize on. Finally, you can use your self-acceptance-inspired list of strengths and weaknesses to remind yourself that you are a complex human being with myriad different aspects.

In the next and final chapter, I will discuss what you have to do to both maintain and extend your philosophy of unconditional self-acceptance.

9

Commit Yourself to Maintaining and Extending Your Developing Self-acceptance Philosophy

I have now taught you all you need to know about unconditional self-acceptance and the skills that you need in order to continue along the path towards greater self-acceptance. I have chosen my words carefully here because no matter how hard you try you will not, in all probability, reach a state of perfect self-acceptance which once attained cannot be lost. Those of you who are perfectionistic and black-and-white in your thinking may react by saying: 'What's the point of even embarking on the journey towards self-acceptance if I cannot hope to achieve it once and for all?' The answer that I usually give is a simple one: 'Working towards greater, but not perfect, self-acceptance is far better than remaining with a philosophy of self-depreciation. Once you accept that this is the reality of the situation you will probably decide to get on with the serious business of maintaining and extending your philosophy of self-acceptance.' To help you do this I offer you the following suggestions.

Keep practising the skills of self-acceptance

The approach to self-acceptance that I have described in this book is skills-oriented in nature. This means that in order to further your journey towards greater self-acceptance you need to practise these skills regularly. You even need to practise these skills when you are feeling good. That's right, your eyes haven't deceived you – I am suggesting that you need to practise the skills that I have outlined in this book even on days when you are feeling good. Why? Because feeling better does not mean that you are in fact deepening your conviction in your self-acceptance philosophy. It may mean that you are facing positive activating events at A in the ABC framework. So what I suggest is that you allocate about twenty minutes a day, five days a week, to practising one or more of the skills that I have taught you in this book, whether you are in a self-depreciating frame of mind or not. This is particularly the case when you are feeling good, since you will be more motivated to use the skills when you are feeling badly about yourself.

Maintaining self-acceptance is akin to maintaining your physical well-being. You wouldn't dream of saying 'Well, I'm feeling OK today so I won't wash myself, clean myself or feed myself.' You take for granted that you need to allocate a certain amount of time per day to activities which help you to maintain your physical well-being. Why, then, is it so strange to accept my point that you need to allocate a certain amount of time per day to activities which may help to maintain your psychological well-being in the area of self-acceptance?

Here is another point that may surprise you. If you are serious about working towards greater self-acceptance then I recommend that you allocate twenty minutes a day, five days a week, to practising the skills of self-acceptance for two years. 'TWO YEARS!!' I hear you exclaim. Yes, two years. In this age of the quick fix, I want to place on record my view that developing self-acceptance takes time and effort. It is not, repeat not, a quick fix. If you feel discouraged by this, adopt the position recommended by Alcoholics Anonymous and take it one day at a time.

Another important point that I want to make to you is that even if you make great strides towards greater self-acceptance, you will still at times begin to depreciate yourself. When this happens you have a choice. Either you use one or more of the skills that I have taught you to identify, challenge and change your rigid demand and self-depreciation belief as soon as you recognize that you are depreciating yourself, or you do nothing, with the result that you will continue to put yourself down. Thus, you cannot realistically stop yourself from depreciating yourself, but you can stop yourself from continuing to put yourself down, by using the skills that I have taught you.

When you commit yourself to regular self-acceptance work, you will be using the range of cognitive, imaginal, emotive and behavioural techniques that I have described in this book. As you do so, it is important that you appreciate one fundamental fact: that you will have to use these techniques regularly before your feelings begin to change. For it is easier to change your beliefs, behaviours and images than it is to effect a fundamental change in your feelings. Accept this basic fact and you will continue to use the techniques that I have taught you even though your feelings haven't yet changed. Demand that your feelings change as soon as you employ these techniques and you will very soon stop using the techniques.

Of all the methods that I have described in this book, perhaps the most important involves you practising your healthy full preferences and self-acceptance beliefs while acting in ways that are consistent with these healthy beliefs. To this end, make this a priority. Use every reasonable opportunity to think healthily and act constructively. Resist your urge to return to habitual ways of behaving when such behaviours are associated with your self-depreciating philosophy. Do shame-attacking exercises regularly, because they are a vivid way of ensuring that you face difficult situations while thinking healthily. As you do so, bear in mind the safeguards that I discussed when carrying out shame-attacking exercises in Chapter 7 (see p. 99).

I have suggested that you regularly use the skills that I have described in this book, but where do I suggest that you start? I suggest that you use the goals that you outlined in Chapter 3 as a framework for change. Map out a sensible plan of action with respect to moving towards your goal. Don't go too slowly, but don't take too much of a jump, either. Use a principle that I have called 'challenging, but not overwhelming', which means doing something that you find difficult, a challenge as it were, but which is not too much for you to do at that time. As you work your way up your hierarchy of difficulty, don't forget to practise your healthy beliefs at every step.

Identifying, challenging and changing your core unhealthy beliefs

So far in this book, I have discussed how to identify, challenge and change the SPECIFIC unhealthy beliefs that underpin your self-deprecia-tion problems. This is a central task, and without it, it is unlikely that you will make much progress along the road to greater self-acceptance.

However, if your problems with self-acceptance are chronic, i.e. you have put yourself down for a long time in a broad range of situations, then it is likely that you also have one or more general or core unhealthy beliefs. A core unhealthy belief constitutes a general belief which in this context takes the form of a general rigid demand and self-depreciation belief that is present across a broad range of situations related to a theme (e.g. disapproval, failure, not being in control). Examples of core unhealthy beliefs that underpin more chronic generalized self-deprecia-tion problems are as follows:

'I must do well at important projects and I'm a failure if I don't.'

'I must be loved and approved by people I deem to be significant and I am worthless if I am not.'

'I must always be strong and show that I am strong and if I don't I am weak and pathetic.'

You will note from the above examples that there is a rigid demand, a self-depreciation statement and a general theme (e.g. doing well, being loved and approved and being strong). The general theme, by definition, must embrace a range of specific situations. Thus if you believe that you must be approved by your teacher alone, but everyone else's approval is desirable, but not essential, to you, you have a specific approval-based unhealthy belief. However, if you believe that you have to be approved by all people in authority to you then you have a more general, core approval-based belief.

You may be wondering at this point, 'When does an unhealthy belief become core?' Unfortunately there is no hard and fast rule about this. What we do know is that core general beliefs vary according to how general they are. Here is an example of how a person's core unhealthy belief may increase in generalness:

- I must be approved by male figures of authority and I am worthless if I am not;
- I must be approved by all figures of authority and I am worthless if I am not;
- I must be approved by all people older than me and I am worthless if I am not;
- I must be approved by everybody and I am worthless if I am not.

It is likely that the more general a core unhealthy belief is, the more it renders the person vulnerable to self-depreciation.

In general, an unhealthy belief is core if it accounts for significant self-depreciation problems in at least three situations related to a particular theme, although it is normally present in a greater number of related situations. Here are a number of ways of identifying core unhealthy beliefs:

1 Look for patterns in your specific ABC analysis. Thus, if you do a number of specific ABC forms you may see recurring patterns in the As about which you put yourself down. If you find a recurring pattern, this is evidence that you may have a core unhealthy belief in this area.
2 List all the situations that you put yourself down in and look for patterns. You might also consult the situations in this regard that I listed in Chapter 3 (see p. 31). Again, if you discover a pattern, you may have a core unhealthy belief in this area.
3 Take your specific unhealthy belief and ask yourself if you put yourself down in similar situations. Once you have identified a specific unhealthy belief (demand and self-depreciation belief) you can check

to see how many situations you hold this belief in. If you find more than three significant situations, then your unhealthy belief may be core.

4 Once you have identified your core unhealthy beliefs, take them one at a time and challenge them using all the techniques that I have taught you in Chapters 5 and 6.

5 List the action tendencies and thinking consequences of your core unhealthy beliefs and list the healthy alternatives to these ways of behaving and thinking.

6 Resolve to act and think in ways that are consistent with your core healthy beliefs and refrain from acting and thinking in ways that are consistent with your core unhealthy beliefs. Do this in a variety of different situations that are relevant to a particular core unhealthy belief. Keep doing this until you can act and think in ways that are consistent with your core healthy belief and can do so without too much difficulty. This step will take a long time, and the more entrenched your core unhealthy belief has been the longer it will take for you to reach this level of competence.

Dealing with lapses

In any programme of constructive personal change, it is virtually certain that you will experience lapses, and this is certainly true as you work to progress along the path to greater self-acceptance. But what is a lapse? I see a lapse as a brief return to a problem state. Unless it is dealt with, you will experience an increasingly greater number of lapses and will eventually experience a relapse, which is what people often refer to as 'going back to square one'. How can you deal with a lapse to prevent it from becoming a relapse? There are three basic things that you need to do here, under the headings below.

Accept yourself for depreciating yourself

When you notice that you are putting yourself down, it would be easy for you to put yourself down for putting yourself down! Stating this in another way, you may bring your self-depreciating attitude to lapses in your progress towards developing self-acceptance. Thus, you may believe that once you know that your rigid demands and self-depreciation beliefs are false, illogical and unhelpful to you then you absolutely must not hold these beliefs any more and you are a stupid person if you do. Challenge this unhealthy belief using the methods that I have already taught you. As you do so it is important to bear in mind a point that I made earlier in this book, that it is not humanly possible to eradicate your tendency to depreciate yourself. This means that at times you will begin to put yourself down. The best you can hope for then is to keep your self-depreciation to a minimum.

Use self-depreciation as a cue for change work

How can you best keep your self-depreciation to a minimum? First, as I said above, by accepting yourself for putting yourself down, and then by using your initial self-depreciation as a cue to work towards self-acceptance using one or more of the methods that I have already taught you. When you recognize that you are depreciating yourself, imagine that this is a yellow traffic light. You are in charge of changing the light to red, by responding to this self-depreciation using some of the techniques that I have discussed in this book, or to green, by doing nothing to counter your self-depreciation and by actively continuing to put yourself down. The more you can change the traffic light to red, the more progress you make towards self-acceptance and the less you will experience lapses.

Develop high frustration tolerance for the slowness and unevenness of significant personal change

Unfortunately there is no quick and easy way to achieve greater self-acceptance. Progress in this area is definitely possible, but it is likely to be fairly slow and uneven. Now, if you demand that such progress must be quick and easy and that you must not experience any setbacks, you will easily become discouraged and stop using the techniques that I have taught you. You will also stop using these methods if you insist that these techniques must be enjoyable. The truth of the matter is that most of you will not find them enjoyable, and after much practice they will become fairly tedious. However, if you accept this grim reality and resolve to keep practising these techniques despite the fact that you do not find them enjoyable and may even find them tedious, then you will gain far more benefit than if you stop using them. In short, remaining on the path towards greater self-acceptance involves you challenging and changing your low frustration tolerance beliefs and acting on a healthier set of high frustration tolerance beliefs. For more on how to do this, I suggest that you consult *Beating the Comfort Trap* (Sheldon Press, 1993) which I wrote with Jack Gordon.

Dealing with unconditional self-depreciation

In Chapter 1, I mentioned that while most people suffer from conditional self-depreciation, meaning that they believe that their worth varies according to changing conditions, some people suffer from unconditional self-depreciation, meaning that they believe that they are worthless and nothing will change this indisputable fact.

As you may imagine, it is much harder to develop self-acceptance when you suffer from unconditional self-depreciation than when your self-depreciation is conditional in nature. This is so because if your worth varies according to changing circumstances, then you acknowledge that you are worthwhile under certain circumstances. Here you are open to the possibility that you can have worth and there is something on which to build. However, when your self-depreciation is unconditional you dismiss the possibility of ever having worth.

Why is your self-depreciation unconditional? How did you come to develop this rigid and wholly negative attitude towards yourself and, more importantly, what can you do about it?

1 Your parents or those who raised you really did not approve of you and treated you as though you were worthless for being alive. In addition, you had no other person who acted as a buffer to this negativity. Here you accepted uncritically the biased unconditional views of others and learned to apply such views to yourself.

   If this is the case, you can still use the methods that I have taught you in the book, but you need to understand that you have accepted without question the unhealthy views of others and practised them until they are second nature. You need to show yourself that your parents were wrong about you, but you were too young to understand that you were wrong and why they were wrong.

   In such cases I have found two additional techniques particularly helpful. First, identify, challenge and change the unhealthy beliefs of your parents (see the book I wrote with Jack Gordon, entitled *How to Cope with Difficult Parents*, Sheldon Press, 1995). Second, use the various versions of the attack–response technique (see pp. 81–88) and respond effectively to those attacks from your parents which you responded to with self-depreciation.

2 You have developed an inhuman set of demands about yourself which you fundamentally believe, but have no chance of reaching. As such you have developed a view that you are worthless just because you are you. Again, you can use all the techniques that I have described in this book AND you can develop a set of high, human standards which you can strive to achieve, and accept yourself when you don't.

3 You believe that you are unconditionally worthless because you have experienced a traumatic event or series of events (usually early in life) and believe that these events, for example, made you irredeemably worthless. Here you may need professional counselling, particularly if

you were sexually abused and/or emotionally abused. You can use the techniques that I outlined here, but do so in conjunction with professional counselling. Consult your GP in the first instance.

4 Finally, you believe you are worthless for no apparent reason. Here you may have a family history of emotional disturbance and may have an inherited tendency to be disturbed yourself, with this expressed most starkly in your attitude of unconditional self-depreciation.

Recognize that for you unconditional self-depreciation is natural but that you can still use the techniques I have described within these pages to develop and strengthen self-acceptance. It will require a lot of practice to change this ingrained way of thinking about yourself, and you will feel very uncomfortable as you do so. But if you tolerate this discomfort and keep working to rip up your rigid demands and self-depreciation beliefs and to replace them with an alternative set of full preferences and self-acceptance beliefs, you will make progress. Persistence, hard work and a willingness to act and think in ways that are consistent with a self-acceptance belief are again important ingredients in the change process. Again, with this type of unconditional self-depreciation you may need professional counselling alongside the work you are doing with yourself which is based on the ideas expressed here. If in doubt, consult your doctor.

Extend your philosophy of unconditional self-acceptance

The final point that I want to make in this book concerns extending your developing philosophy of unconditional self-acceptance. You can do this in a number of different ways. Perhaps the first step you need to take here is to identify and deal with situations where you are particularly vulnerable, in the sense that you would easily depreciate yourself in these situations.

If you want to extend your progress in developing self-acceptance, then it is important that you seek out situations in which you are particularly vulnerable to depreciating yourself and which you would normally go out of your way to avoid, and practise accepting yourself in these situations. Follow the principle of 'challenging, but not overwhelming' as you do this. This means that you seek out situations which are difficult for you to face, but not at that time overwhelming. It is a good idea to construct a hierarchy of such situations, ranging from the easiest to face to the most difficult. Using the emotive-imagery technique that I described on pp. 89–91 is a good preparation for facing the situations in reality. When you face these situations in reality try and ensure that you are actively practising your healthy belief; that your behaviour is functional and does not compensate for implicit self-depreciation; that the way you are thinking about the situation is realistic. If you succeed in making your beliefs, behaviour and thinking healthy, you will get the most out of dealing with your vulnerabilities. If you practise often enough, you may even minimize your vulnerability to depreciating yourself in these situations.

How else can you extend your self-acceptance philosophy? The following are suggestions. You will no doubt have ideas of your own.

1 Ask people what they like and dislike about you and accept yourself for what they say. You may find it particularly difficult to accept yourself when you receive compliments. Watch out for the disqualifying statements you may make in your head, such as 'She is only saying this to be nice', 'He is only saying that because he wants something from me.' These disqualifying statements are often a sign that you are depreciating yourself, so see if you anticipate them, and look for and challenge the underlying demands and self-depreciation beliefs.

2 Teach others the philosophy of self-acceptance. The more you teach these principles to others, the more practice you get at rehearsing them for yourself.

3 Strive to accept others, warts and all. Again, the more you practise other-acceptance, the more likely it is that you will accept yourself, warts and all.

4 Keep practising shame-attacking exercises (see pp. 98–100).

5 Do things that you have always wanted to do, but have held yourself back from doing for self-depreciation reasons.

6 Without harming yourself, admit your faults to others and show them and yourself that you can accept yourself for them.

If you commit yourself to doing such exercises on a regular basis, you will not achieve perfect self-acceptance, but you may become one of the most self-accepting people that you know.

I end this book by wishing you all the best as you continue along the path to self-acceptance. Please let me know how you get on by writing to me c/o Sheldon Press.

Index